NCLEX-PN®:
POWER PRACTICE

NCLEX-PN®:
POWER PRACTICE

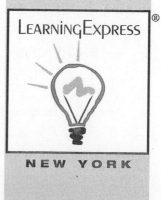

LEARNINGEXPRESS®

NEW YORK

Copyright © 2013 Learning Express, LLC.

All rights reserved under International and Pan American Copyright Conventions.
Published in the United States by LearningExpress, LLC, New York.

Library of Congress Cataloging-in-Publication Data:
NCLEX-PN power practice.
    p. ; cm.
ISBN 978-1-57685-912-4
I. LearningExpress (Organization), publisher.
[DNLM: 1. Nursing, Practical—United States—Examination Questions.   WY 18.2]
RT55
610.7306'93076—dc23

                                                          2013027021

Printed in the United States of America

9 8 7 6 5 4 3 2 1

First Edition

ISBN-13: 978-1-57685-912-4

For more information or to place an order, contact LearningExpress at:
    80 Broad Street
    Suite 400
    New York, NY 10004

Or visit us at:
    www.learningexpressllc.com

CONTENTS

CONTRIBUTORS ▶

Dr. Yvonne Weideman is an assistant professor of nursing at Duquesne University School of Nursing. Her areas of interest are the preparation of students for the NCLEX® exam and the use of innovative technology in the classroom to enhance learning. Dr. Weideman has recently developed a model for integrating theory and content through the use of virtual technology entitled "The Virtual Pregnancy Model."

Dr. Alicia Culleiton is an assistant clinical professor at Duquesne University School of Nursing. She currently teaches doctoral level nursing courses as well as undergraduate NCLEX-RN® preparation courses. Dr. Culleiton earned her BSN from The Catholic University of America, her MSN in nursing administration and nursing education from Indiana University of Pennsylvania, and her doctorate degree from Chatham University. She is published in nursing and educational journals. Her clinical expertise is in emergency/trauma and critical-care nursing, with research interests including student remediation and NCLEX-RN® preparation.

Karen Paraska, PhD, CRNP, is assistant professor of nursing at Duquesne University. She has taught a range of graduate nursing courses, including offerings in advanced practice nursing and research methods, as well as undergraduate courses, including NCLEX-RN® preparation courses. She is coauthor of several referred articles, including "Cognitive impairment associated with adjuvant therapy in breast cancer" for the journal *Psycho-Oncology*.

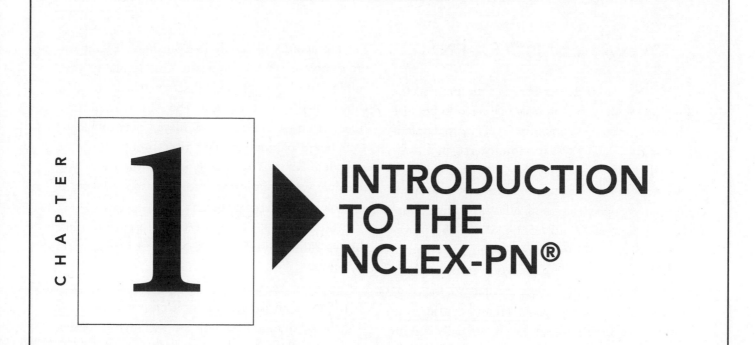

1 ▶ INTRODUCTION TO THE NCLEX-PN®

Congratulations! If you are reading this book, you have graduated or are about to graduate from an accredited licensed practical nurse program and are interested in preparing for the Practical/Vocational Nurses (NCLEX-PN®) examination, which will enable you to become a licensed practical nurse (the term used here for both licensed and vocational practical nurses). One of the most important ways to begin preparing for the NCLEX-PN® is to become familiar with the format of the exam, the process of registering for the exam, what to expect on test day, the subjects the exam covers, and so on. This chapter will help you get started. While the information in this chapter is current as of the date of publication, some details may change. For the most recent information, refer to the official National Council of State Boards of Nursing (NCSBN) NCLEX® website, www.ncsbn.org/nclex.

Overview of NCLEX-PN®

NCLEX-PN® is a computer-based exam that tests the knowledge, skills, and abilities you'll need to practice safely and effectively as an entry-level licensed practical nurse (LPN). The test is administered in a computerized adaptive testing (CAT) format, which allows the computer testing program to evaluate your abilities more effectively and efficiently than more traditional approaches to testing. While the procedure the program uses is complex and will adapt to each individual's abilities, the general principle is fairly simple. With each answer you record, the computer reassesses your competencies and continues to ask additional questions until it is virtually certain that your abilities are above or below the level required.

Given the test's adaptability, the number of questions it asks—anywhere from 85 to 205 items—is different for each individual. Of this number, 25 are pretest questions designed to help test producers develop new types of questions; these are not considered in your assessment. The exam is not divided into sections corresponding to content areas, though it is important that you understand what content areas are covered to help you prepare (see "What Skills Are Tested"). There is a time limit of five hours, no matter what number of questions you are given.

Registering for the Exam

Registration for the NCLEX-PN® is a two-part process: applying for licensure with the board of nursing in the state or territory from which you are seeking your license, and registering for the exam with Pearson VUE, which administers the test. It is advisable to start both phases at once, so that both can proceed simultaneously.

You must meet all your nursing board's requirements for taking the NCLEX-PN® exam. (For a complete list of the boards of nursing and links to their websites, go to www.ncsbn.org/contactbon.htm.) The

nursing board will certify to Pearson VUE that you are eligible to sit for the exam. This results in your Authorization to Test (ATT) letter, which must be shown the day of the exam. The ATT is valid for a time period—from 60 to 365 days—determined by your board of nursing. This time frame cannot be extended. For this reason, it is important that you schedule your appointment for the exam as soon as possible after receiving your ATT.

Step-by-step, the registration process looks like this, as outlined in the "2012 NCLEX® Examination Bulletin":

1. Submit an application for licensure to the board of nursing where you wish to be licensed.
2. Meet all the board of nursing's eligibility requirements to take the NCLEX®.
3. Register for the NCLEX® with Pearson VUE.
4. Receive Acknowledgement of Receipt of Registration from Pearson VUE.
5. The Board of Nursing makes you eligible to take the NCLEX®.
6. Receive Authorization to Test (ATT) letter from Pearson VUE.
7. Schedule your exam with Pearson VUE.

Source: "2013 NCLEX® Examination Bulletin," page 2; available at www.ncsbn.org/2013_NCLEX_Candidate_Bulletin.pdf.

The non-refundable fee to register for the exam is $200. You must also pay fees associated with the licensure application required by your nursing board. The registration is valid for a 365-day period, during which the nursing board will establish your eligibility. If a candidate doesn't meet the board's eligibility requirements within that time period, the registration fee is forfeited.

Failing to appear at the scheduled examination time will also result in the forfeiture of your registration fee and in the invalidation of your ATT, unless you reschedule at least one full business day before your scheduled time. If you don't pass the exam on your first try, you can retest based on a minimum waiting period—45 or 90 days—determined by your state nursing board.

More specific information about registration and scheduling can be found in the "2013 NCLEX® Examination Bulletin," available at www.ncsbn.org/2013_NCLEX_Candidate_Bulletin.pdf. This document and others found at the NCSBN's website should be checked to confirm details, which may change after the publication of this book.

What to Expect at the Test Center

NCLEX-PN® is administered at one of the Pearson Professional Centers (PPCs); there are over 200 of them in the United States with 18 locations outside the United States.

Plan to arrive at least 30 minutes before your test is scheduled to begin. Make sure to bring, in addition to your ATT letter, an acceptable form of personal identification (ID). The only IDs considered acceptable are a U.S. driver's license (Department of Motor Vehicles-issued); U.S. state identification (Department of Motor Vehicles-issued); passport; and U.S. military identification. For test centers outside of the United States, only a passport is acceptable.

In addition to the ID you bring with you, other secure forms of identification will be taken during the check-in process, such as a digital signature and a palm vein scan. For further information on security procedures at the test site, refer to the "2013 NCLEX® Examination Bulletin," available at www.ncsbn.org/2013_NCLEX_Candidate_Bulletin.pdf.

During the Test

The test begins with a brief tutorial, during which you are instructed on how to use the computer you're testing on. As you enter the testing room, the test administrator (TA) will give you an erasable note board and a marker to be used for calculations and note taking. You cannot write on the note board until after the tutorial is finished; writing on it before is considered a serious violation and can result in an incident report and your results being placed on hold. If you need another note board during the test, you can raise your hand and ask the TA to provide you with one. The computer you'll be testing on also has an onscreen calculator to help answer questions requiring calculations.

As mentioned, the time limit for the test is five hours. During this period, there are two optional breaks, one at two hours and another at three and one-half hours; the computer will inform you when these breaks start. You will also be allowed unscheduled breaks, such as those to use the restroom, but all breaks, including those that are scheduled, count against test time.

The testing environment is as standardized as possible to ensure that all candidates complete the exam under the same conditions. Strict controls, therefore, are in effect, such as the audio and video monitoring and recording the restriction against cell phones, pagers, and other electronic devices in the testing room, as well as other personal items such as coats, hats, scarves, gloves, bags, purses, wallets, and watches. See page 8 in the "2013 NCLEX® Examination Bulletin," available at www.ncsbn.org/2013_NCLEX_Candidate_Bulletin.pdf.

What Skills Are Tested?

During your nursing program, much of your study was focused on specific areas of knowledge—such as anatomy and physiology and diseases and pathologies—needed to work as a licensed practical nurse. The key to being an effective LPN, however, is the application of that knowledge. Therefore, the questions—mostly multiple choice, though some are in other formats—are designed to test whether you can apply that knowledge in the safe and effective care of clients as an entry-level PN. The exam, therefore, measures your understanding of the needs of clients you may encounter in practice, as well as your comprehension of the integrated processes critical in addressing these needs.

Client Needs

As mentioned, client needs compose the basic framework for the test plan. Client needs are broken down into four main categories, two of which have subcategories, as is shown in the following table.

CLIENT NEEDS CATEGORIES	PERCENTAGE OF ITEMS IN EACH CATEGORY
Safe and Effective Care Environment	
Coordinated Care	13–19%
Safety and Infection Control	11–17%
Health Promotion and Maintenance	7–13%
Psychosocial Integrity	7–13%
Physiological Integrity	
Basic Care and Comfort	9–15%
Pharmacological Therapies	11–17%
Reduction of Risk Potential	9–15%
Physiological Adaptation	9–15%

Source: "2013 NCLEX® Examination Bulletin," page 13; available at www.ncsbn.org/2013_NCLEX_Candidate_Bulletin.pdf.

These content areas cover the full range of ways that RNs are expected to attend to their clients' needs:

- *Safe and Effective Care Environment: Coordinated Care.* This content area addresses the ways in which the practical nurse should work with the rest of the patient care team to help enhance the safety and effectiveness of the setting in which care is delivered, and the ways that PNs must work to protect clients and healthcare personnel. The skills measured in this content area include, but are not limited to, advance directives, advocacy, informed consent, establishment of priorities, and continuity of care.

- *Safe and Effective Care Environment: Safety and Infection Control.* This content area addresses the ways in which LPNs should work with the rest of the patient care team to protect both clients and healthcare workers from health and environmental hazards. The skills measured in this content area include, but are not limited to, accident, injury, and error preventions; handling hazardous and infectious materials; safe use of equipment; and use of restraints and safety devices.

- *Health Promotion and Maintenance.* This content area addresses the ways in which LPNs should work to incorporate knowledge of growth and development principles and prevention/early-detection strategies into the care of their clients. The skills measured in this content area include, but are not limited to, ante/intra/postpartum and newborn care, developmental stages and transitions, health promotion/disease prevention, lifestyle choices, and data collection techniques.

- *Psychosocial Integrity.* This content area addresses the ways in which LPNs should assist in sustaining and enhancing the emotional, mental, and social well-being of clients as they undergo events causing stress, as well as of clients dealing with acute or long-term mental illness. The skills measured in this content area include, but are not limited to, abuse/neglect, chemical and other dependencies, crisis intervention, end-of-life care, grief and loss, mental health concepts, sensory and perceptual changes, and therapeutic communications and environments.

- *Physiological Integrity: Basic Care and Comfort.* This content area addresses the ways in which LPNs should work to provide comfort to clients, and assist clients in performing activities and meeting expectations of daily living. The skills measured in this content area include, but are not limited to, assistive devices, elimination, mobility and immobility, nutrition and oral hydration, and rest and sleep.

■ *Physiological Integrity: Pharmacological Therapies.* This content area addresses the ways in which LPNs work to provide safe and effective care relating to the administration of medication, and the monitoring of clients receiving parenteral therapies. The skills measured in this content area include, but are not limited to, adverse effects/contraindications/side effects/interactions, dosage calculation, expected actions/outcomes, and medication administration.

■ *Physiological Integrity: Reduction of Risk Potential.* This content area addresses the ways in which LPNs work to reduce the likelihood of complications or problems that arise due to existing conditions, procedures, and treatments. The skills measured in this content area include, but are not limited, to vital signs, diagnostic tests, laboratory values, potential for complications from diagnostic and surgical procedures, and potential changes in body systems (such as cardiovascular, endocrine, gastroenterological, integumentary, musculoskeletal, and neurologic).

■ *Physiological Integrity: Physiological Adaptation.* This content area addresses the ways in which LPNs work to help in the provision of care for patients with acute, chronic, or life-threatening conditions. The skills measured in this content area include, but are not limited to, alterations in body systems, fluid and electrolyte imbalances, medical emergencies, basic pathophysiology, and unexpected response to therapies.

For a more complete explanation and list of examples in each client need category, refer to the the most recent version of the "2011 NCLEX-PN Detailed Test Plan—Candidate," available at www.ncsbn.org/1287.htm.

Integrated Processes

Integrated processes critical to the practice of nursing are also addressed in the questions on the NCLEX-PN® exam. These processes include all the methodologies employed by LPNs in entry-level positions to address their clients' needs. As described in the "2011 NCLEX-PN Detailed Test Plan—Candidate" (available at www.ncsbn.org/1287.htm), they include:

■ *Clinical Problem-Solving Process*—a scientific approach to client care that includes data collection, planning, implementation, and evaluation.

■ *Caring*—interaction of the practical/vocational nurse and client in an atmosphere of mutual respect and trust ... [providing] support and compassion to help achieve desired therapeutic outcomes.

■ *Communication and Documentation*—verbal and nonverbal interactions between the practical/vocational nurse and the client, as well as other members of the healthcare team ... [and] written and/or electronic records that reflect standards of practice and accountability in the provision of care.

■ *Teaching and Learning*—facilitation of the acquisition of knowledge, skills, and attitudes to assist in promoting a change in behavior.

A Note on Guessing

Fast guessing may result in a drastically lowered score. In typical paper-and-pencil tests, and even some administered by a computer, unanswered items are marked wrong. But due to the nature of computer adaptive testing, this strategy is ill-advised, since it will result in the computer program giving candidates easier items, which they may also get wrong if they are guessing and running short on time.

In short, rapid guessing should be avoided. You should simply maintain a steady pace—allotting approximately one to two minutes on each item. Stay focused and carefully read each item before answering.

Exam Results

Examination results are mailed by the board of nursing to the candidate approximately one month after the test. If you haven't received them after four weeks, you should contact your board of nursing, not Pearson VUE. Unofficial results are available within 48 hours through Quick Results Service for a small fee, if your board of nursing participates in the program.

To ensure quality and accuracy, the results are scored twice—once by the computer and a second time after the computer results are transmitted to Pearson VUE's central office. And even though the computer obtains the candidate's results, this information is not available to the test center's staff.

If you fail the exam, you will receive a Candidate Performance Report (CPR) from your nursing board. In addition to notifying the candidate of the unacceptable performance on the test, the CPR includes information about the number of items administered and the candidate's relative strengths and weaknesses vis-à-vis the test plan. With this information, you will be guided in your preparation for retaking the exam. As mentioned, the retake waiting period depends on your board of nursing, and will be a minimum of 45 or 90 days between each exam.

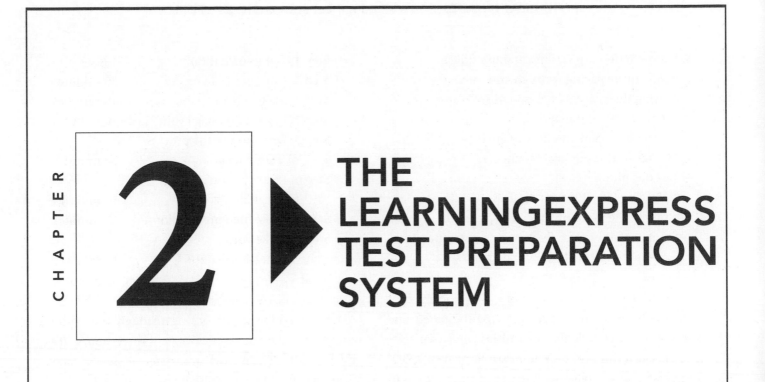

2 ▶ THE LEARNINGEXPRESS TEST PREPARATION SYSTEM

t takes significant preparation to score well on any exam, and NCLEX-PN® is no exception. The Learning-Express Test Preparation System, developed by experts exclusively for LearningExpress, offers a number of strategies designed to facilitate the development of the skills, disciplines, and attitudes necessary for success.

Preparing for and attaining a passing score on the NCLEX-PN® exam requires surmounting an assortment of obstacles. While some may prove more troublesome than others, all of them carry the potential to hinder your performance, and negatively affect your scores. Here are some examples:

- lack of familiarity with the exam format
- paralyzing test anxiety
- leaving preparation to the last minute
- not preparing at all

- failure to develop vital test-taking skills:
  - effectively pacing through an exam
  - using the process of elimination to answer questions accurately
  - knowing when and how to guess
- mental and/or physical fatigue
- Test day blunders:
  - arriving late at the testing facility
  - taking the exam on an empty stomach
  - not accounting for fluctuations in temperature at the testing facility

The common thread among these obstacles is control. While a host of pressing, unanticipated, and sometimes unavoidable difficulties may frustrate your preparation, there remain some proven, effective strategies for placing yourself in the best possible position on exam day. These strategies can significantly improve your level of comfort with the exam, offering you not only the confidence you'll need, but also, and perhaps most importantly, a higher test score.

The LearningExpress Test Preparation System helps to put you in greater control. Separated into nine steps, the system heightens your confidence level by helping you understand both the exam and your own particular set of test-taking strengths and weaknesses. It helps you structure a study plan, practice a number of effective test-taking skills, and avoid mental and physical fatigue on exam day. Each step is accompanied by an activity.

While the following list suggests an approximate time for the completion of each step, these are only guidelines for your initial introduction. The regular practice of a number of them may require a more substantial time commitment. It may also be necessary and helpful to return to one or more of them throughout the course of your preparation.

Step 1.	Get information.	1 hour
Step 2.	Conquer test anxiety.	20 minutes
Step 3.	Make a plan.	20 minutes
Step 4.	Learn to manage your time.	10 minutes
Step 5.	Learn to use the process of elimination.	20 minutes
Step 6.	Reach your peak performance zone.	10 minutes
Step 7.	Make final preparations.	10 minutes
Step 8.	Make your preparations count.	10 minutes
Total		2 hours, 30 minutes

We estimate that working through the entire system will take you approximately three hours. It's perfectly okay if you work at a faster or slower pace. It's up to you to decide whether you should set aside a whole afternoon or evening to work through the LearningExpress Test Preparation System in one sitting, or break it up and do just one or two steps a day for the next several days.

Step 1: Get Information

Time to complete: 1 hour
Activities: Read the introduction to this book.

Knowing more about an exam can often make it appear less daunting. The first step in the LearningExpress Test Preparation System is to determine everything you can about the type of information you will be expected to know on the NCLEX-PN®, as well as how your knowledge will be assessed.

What You Should Find Out

Knowing the details will help you study efficiently and help you feel a sense of control. Here's a list of things you might want to find out:

- What skills are tested?
- How many sections are on the exam?
- How many questions are in each section?
- How much time is allotted for each section?
- How is the exam scored, and is there a penalty for guessing/wrong answers?
- Is the test computerized or will you have an exam booklet?
- Will you be given scratch paper to write on?

You will find answers to these questions in Chapter 1 of this book and on the NCSBN's NCLEX-PN® website, www.ncsbn.org.

Step 2: Conquer Test Anxiety

Time to complete: 20 minutes
Activity: Take the Test Stress Quiz.

Now that you know what's on the test, the next step is to address one of the biggest obstacles to success: *test anxiety*. Test anxiety may not only impair your performance on the exam itself, but it can also keep you from preparing properly. In Step 2, you will learn stress management techniques that will help you succeed on your exam. Practicing these techniques as you work through the activities in this book will help them become second nature to you by exam day.

Combating Test Anxiety

A little test anxiety is a good thing. Everyone gets nervous before a big exam—and if that nervousness motivates you to prepare thoroughly, so much the better. Many athletes report pregame jitters, which they are able to harness to help them perform at their peak. Stop here and answer the questions on the Test Stress Quiz that follows to determine your level of test anxiety.

Stress Management before the Exam

If you feel your level of anxiety is getting the best of you in the weeks before the exam, here are things you can do to bring the level down:

- **Prepare.** There's nothing like knowing what to expect to put you in control of test anxiety. That's why you're reading this book. Use it faithfully, and you will be ready on test day.
- **Practice self-confidence.** A positive attitude is a great way to combat test anxiety. Stand in front of the mirror and say to your reflection, "I'm prepared. I'm confident. I'm going to ace this exam. I know I can do it." As soon as negative thoughts creep in, drown them out with these positive affirmations. If you hear them often enough, and you use the LearningExpress method to study for NCLEX-PN®, they will be true.
- **Fight negative messages.** Every time someone talks to you about how hard the exam is or says it's difficult to pass, think about your self-confidence messages. If the someone with the negative messages is you—you're telling yourself you don't do well on exams, that you just can't do this—don't listen. Repeat self-confidence messages.
- **Visualize.** Visualizing success can help make it happen, and it reminds you of why you're doing all this work in preparing for the exam. Imagine yourself in your first day of classes or beginning the first day of your dream job.
- **Exercise.** Physical activity helps calm your body and focus your mind. Besides, being in good physical shape can actually help you do well on the exam. Go for a run, lift weights, go swimming—and exercise regularly.

You need to worry about test anxiety only if it is extreme enough to impair your performance. The following questionnaire provides a diagnosis of your level of test anxiety. In the blank before each statement, write the number that most accurately describes your experience.

0 = Never
1 = Once or twice
2 = Sometimes
3 = Often

____ I have gotten so nervous before an exam that I simply put down the books and didn't study for it.

____ I have experienced disabling physical symptoms such as vomiting and severe headaches because I was nervous about an exam.

____ I have simply not showed up for an exam because I was scared to take it.

____ I have experienced dizziness and disorientation while taking an exam.

____ I have had trouble filling in the little circles because my hands were shaking too hard.

____ I have failed an exam because I was too nervous to complete it.

____ **Total: Add up the numbers in the blanks.**

Your Test Stress Score

Here are the steps you should take, depending on your score. If you scored:

- **Below 3,** your level of test anxiety is nothing to worry about; it's probably just enough to give you that extra edge.

- **Between 3 and 6,** your test anxiety may be enough to impair your performance, and you should practice the stress-management techniques in this section to try to bring your test anxiety down to manageable levels.

- **Above 6,** your level of test anxiety is a serious concern. In addition to practicing the stress management techniques listed in this section, you may want to seek additional, personal help. Call your community college and ask for the academic counselor or ask the counselor at your nursing school. Tell the counselor that you have a level of test anxiety that sometimes keeps you from being able to take the exam. The counselor may be willing to help you or may suggest someone else you should talk to.

Stress Management on Test Day

There are several ways you can bring down your level of test stress and anxiety on test day. They'll work best if you practice them in the weeks before the exam, so you know which ones work best for you.

- **Breathe deeply.** Take a deep breath in while you count to five. Hold it for a count of one, and then let it out on a count of five. Repeat several times.
- **Move your body.** Try rolling your head in a circle. Rotate your shoulders. Shake your hands from the wrist.
- **Visualize again.** Think of the place where you are most relaxed: lying on the beach in the sun, walking through the park, or wherever relaxes you. Now, close your eyes and imagine you're actually there. If you practice in advance, you will find that you need only a few seconds of this exercise to experience a significant increase in your sense of relaxation and well-being.

When anxiety threatens to overwhelm you during the test, there are still things you can do to manage your stress level:

- **Repeat your self-confidence messages.** You should have them memorized by now. Say them quietly to yourself, and believe them!
- **Visualize one more time.** This time, visualize yourself moving smoothly and quickly through the exam, answering every question correctly, and finishing just before time is up. Like most visualization techniques, this one works best if you've practiced it ahead of time.
- **Find an easy question.** Skim over the questions until you find an easy one, and then answer it. Getting even one question answered correctly gets you into the test-taking groove.

- **Take a mental break.** Everyone loses concentration once in a while during a long exam. It's normal, so you shouldn't worry about it. Instead, accept what has happened. Say to yourself, "Hey, I lost it there for a minute. My brain is taking a break." Close your eyes and do some deep breathing for a few seconds. Then go back to work.

Try these techniques ahead of time and see whether they work for you!

Step 3: Make a Plan

Time to complete: 20 minutes
Activity: Construct a study plan.

There is no substitute for careful preparation and practice over time. So the most important thing you can do to better prepare yourself for your exam is to create a study plan or schedule and then follow it. This will help you avoid cramming at the last minute, which is an ineffective study technique that will only add to your anxiety.

Once you make your plan, make a commitment to follow it. Set aside at least 30 minutes every day for studying and practice. This will do more good than two hours crammed into a Saturday. If you have months before the test, you're lucky. Don't put off your studying until the week before. Start now. Even 10 minutes on weekdays, with half an hour or more on weekends, can make a big difference in your score.

Step 4: Learn to Manage Your Time

Time to complete: 10 minutes to read, many hours of practice
Activities: Practice these strategies as you take the sample exams.

Steps 4, 5, and 6 of the LearningExpress Test Preparation System put you in charge of your NCLEX-PN® experience by showing you test-taking strategies that work. Practice these strategies as you take the practice exams in this book and online. Then, you will be ready to use them on test day.

First, you will take control of your time on NCLEX-PN®. Start by understanding the format of the test. Refer to Chapter 1 to review this information; in particular, make sure you understand the way the computerized adaptive testing (CAT) works.

You will want to practice using your time wisely on the practice tests, while trying to avoid making mistakes while working quickly.

- **Listen carefully to directions.** By the time you get to the test, you should know how it works. But listen carefully in case something has changed.
- **Pace yourself.** Glance at your watch every few minutes to ensure that you are not taking much more than one to two minutes on each question.
- **Keep moving.** Don't spend too much time on one question. If you don't know the answer, skip the question and move on. Mark the question for review and come back to it later, if possible.
- **Don't rush.** You should keep moving, but rushing won't help. Try to keep calm and work methodically and quickly.

Step 5: Learn to Use the Process of Elimination

Time to complete: 20 minutes
Activity: Complete worksheet on the process of elimination.

After time management, the next most important tool for taking control of your test is using the process of elimination wisely. It's standard test-taking wisdom that you should always read all the answer choices before choosing your answer. This helps you find the right answer by eliminating wrong answer choices. Consider the following question. Although it is not the type of question you will see on NCLEX-PN®, the mental process that you use will be the same.

> **Sentence 6:** I would like to be considered for the assistant manager position in your company my previous work experience is a good match for the job requirements posted.
> Which correction should be made to sentence 6?
> **a.** Insert *Although* before *I*.
> **b.** Insert a question mark after *company*.
> **c.** Insert a semicolon and *however* before *my*.
> **d.** Insert a period after *company* and capitalize *my*.
> **e.** No corrections are necessary.

If you happen to know that sentence 6 is a run-on sentence, and you know how to correct it, you don't need to use the process of elimination. But let's assume that, like some people, you don't. So, you look at the answer choices. *Although* sure doesn't sound like a good choice, because it would change the meaning of the sentence. So, you eliminate choice **a**, and now you only have four answer choices to deal with.

Write **a** on your note board with an X through or beside it. Move on to the other answer choices.

If you know that the first part of the sentence does not ask a question, you can eliminate choice **b** as a possible answer. Write **b** on your note board with an X through or beside it. Choice **c**, inserting a semicolon, could create a pause in an otherwise long sentence, but inserting the word *however* might not be correct. If you're not sure whether this answer is correct, write **c** on your note board with a question mark beside it, meaning "well, maybe."

Choice **d** would separate a very long sentence into two shorter sentences, and it would not change the meaning. It could work, so write **d** on your note board with a check mark beside it, meaning "good answer." Choice **e** means that the sentence is fine like it is and doesn't need any changes. The sentence could make sense as it is, but it is definitely long. Is this the best way to write the sentence? If you're not sure, write **e** on your note board with a question mark beside it.

Now, your note board looks like this:

X **a.**
X **b.**
? **c.**
✓ **d.**
? **e.**

You've got just one check mark, for a good answer, **d**. If you're pressed for time, you should simply select choice **d**. If you've got the time to be extra careful, you could compare your check mark answer to your question mark answers to make sure that it's better. (It is: Sentence 6 is a run-on, and should be separated into two shorter, complete sentences.)

It's good to have a system for marking good, bad, and maybe answers. We recommend using this one:

X = bad
✓ = good
? = maybe

If you don't like these marks, devise your own system. Just make sure you do it long before exam day—while you're working through the practice tests in this book and online—so you won't have to worry about it during the exam.

Even when you think you're absolutely clueless about a question, you can use the process of elimination to get rid of one answer choice. By doing so, you're better prepared to make an educated guess. Often, the process of elimination allows you to get down to only two possible right answers. Nevertheless, as explained in Chapter 1, rapid guessing is a strategy that should be avoided in the NCLEX-PN®. It will result in the computer program giving candidates easier items, which you may also get wrong if you are guessing and running short on time.

Try using your powers of elimination on the following questions. The answer explanations show one possible way you might use the process to arrive at the right answer.

Step 6: Reach Your Peak Performance Zone

Time to complete: 10 minutes to read, weeks to complete!
Activity: Complete the Physical Preparation Checklist.

Physical and mental fatigue can significantly hinder your ability to perform not only as you prepare, but also on the day of the exam. Poor diet choices can hinder you, as well. Drastic changes to your existing daily routine may cause a disruption too great to be helpful, but modest, calculated alterations in your level of physical activity, the quality of your diet, and the amount and regularity of your rest can enhance your studies and your performance on the exam.

USING THE PROCESS OF ELIMINATION

Use the process of elimination to answer the following questions.

1. Ilsa is as old as Meghan will be in five years. The difference between Ed's age and Meghan's age is twice the difference between Ilsa's age and Meghan's age. Ed is 29. How old is Ilsa?
   a. 4
   b. 10
   c. 19
   d. 24

2. "All drivers of commercial vehicles must carry a valid commercial driver's license whenever operating a commercial vehicle."
   According to this sentence, which of the following people need NOT carry a commercial driver's license?
   a. a truck driver idling his engine while waiting to be directed to a loading dock
   b. a bus operator backing her bus out of the way of another bus in the bus lot
   c. a taxi driver driving his personal car to the grocery store
   d. a limousine driver taking the limousine to her home after dropping off her last passenger of the evening

3. Smoking tobacco has been linked to
   a. increased risk of stroke and heart attack.
   b. all forms of respiratory disease.
   c. increasing mortality rates over the past 10 years.
   d. juvenile delinquency.

4. Which of the following words is spelled correctly?
   a. incorrigible
   b. outragous
   c. domestickated
   d. understandible

Answers

Here are the answers, as well as some suggestions as to how you might have used the process of elimination to find them.

1. d. You should have eliminated choice a right off the bat. Ilsa can't be four years old if Meghan is going to be Ilsa's age in five years. The best way to eliminate other answer choices is to try plugging them into the information given in the problem. For instance, for choice **b**, if Ilsa is 10, then Meghan must be 5. The difference between their ages is 5. The difference between Ed's age, 29, and Meghan's age, 5, is 24. Is 24 two times 5? No. Then choice **b** is wrong. You could eliminate choice **c** in the same way and be left with choice **d**.

2. c. Note the word not in the question, and go through the answers one by one. Is the truck driver in choice **a** "operating a commercial vehicle"? Yes, idling counts as "operating," so he needs to have a commercial driver's license. Likewise, the bus operator in choice **b** is operating a commercial vehicle; the question doesn't say the operator has to be on the street. The limo driver in choice **d** is operating a commercial vehicle, even if it doesn't have a passenger in it. However, the driver in choice **c** is not operating a commercial vehicle, but his own private car.

3. a. You could eliminate choice **b** simply because of the presence of the word *all*. Such absolutes hardly ever appear in correct answer choices. Choice **c** looks attractive until you think a little about what you know—aren't fewer people smoking these days, rather than more? So how could smoking be responsible for a higher mortality rate? (If you didn't know that mortality rate means the rate at which people die, you might keep this choice as a possibility, but you would still be able to eliminate two answers and have only two to choose from.) And choice **d** is plain silly, so you could eliminate that one, too. You are left with the correct choice, **a**.

4. a. How you used the process of elimination here depends on which words you recognized as being spelled incorrectly. If you knew that the correct spellings were *outrageous*, *domesticated*, and *understandable*, then you would be home free. Surely you knew that at least one of those words was wrong in the question!

Exercise

If you are already engaged in a regular program of physical activity, resist allowing the pressure of the approaching exam to alter this routine. If you are not, and have not been engaged in regular physical activity, it may be helpful to begin during your preparations. Speak with someone knowledgeable about such matters to design a regimen suited to your particular circumstances and needs. Whatever its form, try to keep it a regular part of your preparation as the exam approaches.

Diet

A balanced diet will help you achieve peak performance. Limit your caffeine and junk food intake as you continue on your preparation journey. Eat plenty

The following are ten really hard questions. You are not supposed to know the answers. Rather, this is an assessment of your ability to guess when you don't have a clue. Read each question carefully, as if you were expected to answer it. If you have any knowledge of the subject, use that knowledge to help you eliminate wrong answer choices.

1. September 7 is Independence Day in
   a. India.
   b. Costa Rica.
   c. Brazil.
   d. Australia.

2. Which of the following is the formula for determining the momentum of an object?
   a. $p = MV$
   b. $F = ma$
   c. $P = IV$
   d. $E = mc^2$

3. Because of the expansion of the universe, the stars and other celestial bodies are all moving away from each other. This phenomenon is known as
   a. Newton's first law.
   b. the big bang.
   c. gravitational collapse.
   d. Hubble flow.

4. American author Gertrude Stein was born in
   a. 1713.
   b. 1830.
   c. 1874.
   d. 1901.

5. Which of the following is NOT one of the Five Classics attributed to Confucius?
   a. *I Ching*
   b. *Book of Holiness*
   c. *Spring and Autumn Annals*
   d. *Book of History*

6. The religious and philosophical doctrine that holds that the universe is constantly in a struggle between good and evil is known as
   a. Pelagianism.
   b. Manichaeanism.
   c. neo-Hegelianism.
   d. Epicureanism.

7. The third Chief Justice of the U.S. Supreme Court was
   a. John Blair.
   b. William Cushing.
   c. James Wilson.
   d. John Jay.

8. Which of the following is the poisonous portion of a daffodil?
   a. the bulb
   b. the leaves
   c. the stem
   d. the flowers

9. The winner of the Masters golf tournament in 1953 was
   a. Sam Snead.
   b. Cary Middlecoff.
   c. Arnold Palmer.
   d. Ben Hogan.

10. The state with the highest per capita personal income in 1980 was
    a. Alaska.
    b. Connecticut.
    c. New York.
    d. Texas.

Answers

Check your answers against the following correct answers.

1. c.
2. a.
3. d.
4. c.
5. b.
6. b.
7. b.
8. a.
9. d.
10. a.

How Did You Do?

You may have simply gotten lucky and actually known the answer to one or two questions. In addition, your guessing was probably more successful if you were able to use the process of elimination on any of the questions. Maybe you didn't know who the third Chief Justice was (question 7), but you knew that John Jay was the first. In that case, you would have eliminated choice **d** and, therefore, improved your odds of guessing right from one in four to one in three.

According to probability, you should get two-and-a-half answers correct, so getting either two or three right would be average. If you got four or more right, you may be a really terrific guesser. If you got one or none right, you may be a really bad guesser.

Keep in mind, though, that this is only a small sample. You should continue to keep track of your guessing ability as you work through the sample questions in this book. Circle the numbers of questions you guess on as you make your guess; or, if you don't have time while you take the practice tests, go back afterward and try to remember which questions you guessed at. Remember, on a test with four answer choices, your chance of guessing correctly is one in four. So keep a separate "guessing" score for each exam. How many questions did you guess on? How many did you get right? If the number you got right is at least one-fourth of the number of questions you guessed on, you are at least an average guesser—maybe better—and you should always go ahead and guess on the real exam. If the number you got right is significantly lower than one-fourth of the number you guessed on, you would be safe in guessing anyway, but maybe you would feel more comfortable if you guessed only selectively, when you can eliminate a wrong answer or at least have a good feeling about one of the answer choices.

Remember, even if you are a play-it-safe person with lousy intuition, you are still safe guessing every time.

---

of fruits and vegetables, along with lean proteins and complex carbohydrates. Foods that are high in lecithin (an amino acid), such as fish and beans, are especially good brain foods.

Your diet is also a matter that is particular to you, so any major alterations to it should be discussed with a person with expert knowledge of nutrition.

Rest

For your brain and body to function at optimal levels, they must have an adequate amount of rest. It is important to determine what an adequate amount of rest is for you. Determine how much rest you need to feel at your sharpest and most alert, and make an effort to get that amount regularly as the exam approaches and particularly on the night before the exam.

It may help to record your efforts. What follows is a Physical Preparation Checklist for the week prior to the exam; you may find its use helpful for staying on track.

PHYSICAL PREPARATION CHECKLIST

For the week before the test, record the type and duration of your physical exercise, your food consumption for each day, and the number of hours you slept.

Exam minus 7 days

Exercise: _____ for _____ minutes

Breakfast: _____

Lunch: _____

Dinner: _____

Snacks: _____

Sleep: _____

Exam minus 6 days

Exercise: _____ for _____ minutes

Breakfast: _____

Lunch: _____

Dinner: _____

Snacks: _____

Sleep: _____

Exam minus 5 days

Exercise: _____ for _____ minutes

Breakfast: _____

Lunch: _____

Dinner: _____

Snacks: _____

Sleep: _____

Exam minus 4 days

Exercise: _____ for _____ minutes

Breakfast: _____

Lunch: _____

Dinner: _____

Snacks: _____

Sleep: _____

Exam minus 3 days

Exercise: _____ for _____ minutes

Breakfast: _____

Lunch: _____

Dinner: _____

Snacks: _____

Sleep: _____

Exam minus 2 days

Exercise: _____ for _____ minutes

Breakfast: _____

Lunch: _____

Dinner: _____

Snacks: _____

Sleep: _____

Exam minus 1 day

Exercise: _____ for _____ minutes

Breakfast: _____

Lunch: _____

Dinner: _____

Snacks: _____

Sleep: _____

Physical Preparation Checklist

In the week leading up to the test, you may be so involved with studying (and, unfortunately, stress) that you neglect to treat your body kindly. The worksheet on the following page will help you stay on track.

For each day of the week before the test, write down what physical exercise you engaged in and for how long and what you ate for each meal. Remember, you're trying for at least half an hour of exercise every other day (preferably every day) and a balanced diet that is light on junk food. These practices are key to your body and brain working at their peak.

Step 7: Make Final Preparations

Time to complete: 10 minutes to read; time to complete will vary
Activity: Complete the Final Preparations worksheet.

You're in control of your mind and body; you're in charge of test anxiety, your preparation, and your test-taking strategies. Now, it's time to take charge of external factors, like the testing site and the materials you need to take the test.

Find Out Where the Exam Is and Make a Trial Run

Make sure you know exactly when and where your test is being held. Do you know how to get to the exam site? Do you know how long it will take to get there? If not, make a trial run if possible, preferably on the same day of the week at the same time of day. On the Final Preparations worksheet, make note of the amount of time it will take you to get to the test site. Plan on arriving at least 30 to 45 minutes early so you can get the lay of the land, use the bathroom, and calm down. Then figure out how early you will have

to get up that morning, and make sure you get up that early every day for a week before the test.

Gather Your Materials

Make sure you have all the materials that will be required at the testing facility. Whether it's an admission ticket, two forms of ID, pencils, pens, calculators, a watch, or any other item that may be necessary, make sure you have put it aside. It's preferable to put them all aside together.

Arrange your clothes the evening before the exam. Dress in layers so that you can adjust readily to the temperature of the exam room.

Fuel Appropriately

Decide on a meal to eat in the time before your exam. Taking the exam on an empty stomach is something to avoid, particularly if it is an exam that spans several hours. Eating poorly and feeling lethargic are also to be avoided. Decide on a meal that will sate your hunger without adverse effect.

Final Preparations

To help get organized, a Final Preparations worksheet is included here.

Step 8: Make Your Preparations Count

Time to complete: 10 minutes, plus test-taking time
Activity: Ace the NCLEX-PN®!

Fast forward to test day. You're ready. You made a study plan and followed through. You practiced your test-taking strategies while working through this book. You're in control of your physical, mental, and emotional state. You know when and where to show up and what to bring with you. In other words, you're well prepared!

When you're finished with the test, you will have earned a reward. Plan a celebration. Call up your friends and plan a party, have a nice dinner with your family, or pick out a movie to see—whatever your heart desires.

And then do it. Go into the test full of confidence, armed with test-taking strategies you've practiced until they're second nature. You're in control of yourself, your environment, and your performance on the exam. You're ready to succeed. So do it. And look forward to your future as someone who has passed the NCLEX-PN®!

Getting to the exam site:

Exam date: _____

Location of exam site: _____

Do I know how to get to the exam site?   Yes ___   No ___   (If no, make a trial run.)

Time it will take to get to the exam site: _____

Departure time: _____

Things to Lay Out the Night Before

Clothes I will wear   ___

Sweater/jacket   ___

Watch   ___

Photo ID   ___

Four #2 pencils   ___

Other Things to Bring/Remember

_____   _____

_____   _____

_____   _____

_____   _____

3 ▶ NCLEX-PN®
PRACTICE TEST 1

This exam has been designed to test your understanding of the content included on the National Council Licensure Examination for Licensed Practical/Vocational Nurses (NCLEX-PN®). Becoming comfortable with the exam format and logistics will help you be more relaxed when it comes to actually sitting for the test, enabling you to perform at your best.

The actual NCLEX-PN® exam is computer adaptive, which means all examinees will have a different number of test questions depending on how many and what types of questions they answer correctly and incorrectly. All test takers must answer a minimum of 85 items, and the maximum number of items that the candidate may answer is 205 during the allotted five-hour time period. This LearningExpress practice exam has 165 questions, and you should allow yourself four hours to complete it.

After you have completed the exam, look at the answer key to read the rationale for both the correct and incorrect choices, as well as the sources of the information. It is recommended that you utilize the sources to thoroughly review information that was problematic for you. Because the NCLEX-PN® examination is graded on a sliding scale that is based on the difficulty of each particular exam, we are unable to predict how many correct answers would equate to an actual passing grade on this practice exam.

Completion of this exam represents the culmination of extensive test preparation. You have worked very hard to review the information from your NCLEX-PN® curriculum, and now it is your time to shine. Good luck!

Practice Test 1 Answer Sheet

#						#						#				
1.	ⓐ	ⓑ	ⓒ	ⓓ		56.	ⓐ	ⓑ	ⓒ	ⓓ		111.	ⓐ	ⓑ	ⓒ	ⓓ
2.	ⓐ	ⓑ	ⓒ	ⓓ		57.	ⓐ	ⓑ	ⓒ	ⓓ		112.	ⓐ	ⓑ	ⓒ	ⓓ
3.	ⓐ	ⓑ	ⓒ	ⓓ		58.	ⓐ	ⓑ	ⓒ	ⓓ		113.	ⓐ	ⓑ	ⓒ	ⓓ
4.	ⓐ	ⓑ	ⓒ	ⓓ		59.	ⓐ	ⓑ	ⓒ	ⓓ		114.	ⓐ	ⓑ	ⓒ	ⓓ
5.	ⓐ	ⓑ	ⓒ	ⓓ		60.	ⓐ	ⓑ	ⓒ	ⓓ		115.	ⓐ	ⓑ	ⓒ	ⓓ
6.	ⓐ	ⓑ	ⓒ	ⓓ		61.	_____					116.	ⓐ	ⓑ	ⓒ	ⓓ
7.	ⓐ	ⓑ	ⓒ	ⓓ		62.	ⓐ	ⓑ	ⓒ	ⓓ		117.	ⓐ	ⓑ	ⓒ	ⓓ
8.	ⓐ	ⓑ	ⓒ	ⓓ		63.	ⓐ	ⓑ	ⓒ	ⓓ		118.	ⓐ	ⓑ	ⓒ	ⓓ
9.	ⓐ	ⓑ	ⓒ	ⓓ		64.	_____					119.	ⓐ	ⓑ	ⓒ	ⓓ
10.	ⓐ	ⓑ	ⓒ	ⓓ		65.	ⓐ	ⓑ	ⓒ	ⓓ		120.	ⓐ	ⓑ	ⓒ	ⓓ
11.	ⓐ	ⓑ	ⓒ	ⓓ		66.	ⓐ	ⓑ	ⓒ	ⓓ		121.	ⓐ	ⓑ	ⓒ	ⓓ
12.	ⓐ	ⓑ	ⓒ	ⓓ		67.	ⓐ	ⓑ	ⓒ	ⓓ		122.	ⓐ	ⓑ	ⓒ	ⓓ
13.	ⓐ	ⓑ	ⓒ	ⓓ		68.	ⓐ	ⓑ	ⓒ	ⓓ		123.	ⓐ	ⓑ	ⓒ	ⓓ
14.	ⓐ	ⓑ	ⓒ	ⓓ		69.	ⓐ	ⓑ	ⓒ	ⓓ		124.	ⓐ	ⓑ	ⓒ	ⓓ
15.	ⓐ	ⓑ	ⓒ	ⓓ		70.	ⓐ	ⓑ	ⓒ	ⓓ		125.	ⓐ	ⓑ	ⓒ	ⓓ
16.	ⓐ	ⓑ	ⓒ	ⓓ		71.	ⓐ	ⓑ	ⓒ	ⓓ		126.	ⓐ	ⓑ	ⓒ	ⓓ
17.	ⓐ	ⓑ	ⓒ	ⓓ		72.	ⓐ	ⓑ	ⓒ	ⓓ		127.	ⓐ	ⓑ	ⓒ	ⓓ
18.	ⓐ	ⓑ	ⓒ	ⓓ		73.	ⓐ	ⓑ	ⓒ	ⓓ		128.	ⓐ	ⓑ	ⓒ	ⓓ
19.	ⓐ	ⓑ	ⓒ	ⓓ		74.	ⓐ	ⓑ	ⓒ	ⓓ		129.	ⓐ	ⓑ	ⓒ	ⓓ
20.	ⓐ	ⓑ	ⓒ	ⓓ		75.	ⓐ	ⓑ	ⓒ	ⓓ		130.	ⓐ	ⓑ	ⓒ	ⓓ
21.	ⓐ	ⓑ	ⓒ	ⓓ		76.	ⓐ	ⓑ	ⓒ	ⓓ		131.	ⓐ	ⓑ	ⓒ	ⓓ
22.	ⓐ	ⓑ	ⓒ	ⓓ		77.	ⓐ	ⓑ	ⓒ	ⓓ		132.	ⓐ	ⓑ	ⓒ	ⓓ
23.	ⓐ	ⓑ	ⓒ	ⓓ		78.	ⓐ	ⓑ	ⓒ	ⓓ		133.	ⓐ	ⓑ	ⓒ	ⓓ
24.	ⓐ	ⓑ	ⓒ	ⓓ		79.	ⓐ	ⓑ	ⓒ	ⓓ		134.	ⓐ	ⓑ	ⓒ	ⓓ
25.	ⓐ	ⓑ	ⓒ	ⓓ		80.	ⓐ	ⓑ	ⓒ	ⓓ		135.	ⓐ	ⓑ	ⓒ	ⓓ
26.	ⓐ	ⓑ	ⓒ	ⓓ		81.	ⓐ	ⓑ	ⓒ	ⓓ		136.	ⓐ	ⓑ	ⓒ	ⓓ
27.	ⓐ	ⓑ	ⓒ	ⓓ		82.	ⓐ	ⓑ	ⓒ	ⓓ		137.	ⓐ	ⓑ	ⓒ	ⓓ
28.	_____					83.	ⓐ	ⓑ	ⓒ	ⓓ		138.	ⓐ	ⓑ	ⓒ	ⓓ
29.	ⓐ	ⓑ	ⓒ	ⓓ		84.	_____					139.	ⓐ	ⓑ	ⓒ	ⓓ
30.	ⓐ	ⓑ	ⓒ	ⓓ		85.	ⓐ	ⓑ	ⓒ	ⓓ		140.	ⓐ	ⓑ	ⓒ	ⓓ
31.	ⓐ	ⓑ	ⓒ	ⓓ		86.	ⓐ	ⓑ	ⓒ	ⓓ		141.	ⓐ	ⓑ	ⓒ	ⓓ
32.	ⓐ	ⓑ	ⓒ	ⓓ		87.	ⓐ	ⓑ	ⓒ	ⓓ		142.	_____			
33.	ⓐ	ⓑ	ⓒ	ⓓ		88.	ⓐ	ⓑ	ⓒ	ⓓ		143.	ⓐ	ⓑ	ⓒ	ⓓ
34.	ⓐ	ⓑ	ⓒ	ⓓ		89.	ⓐ	ⓑ	ⓒ	ⓓ		144.	ⓐ	ⓑ	ⓒ	ⓓ
35.	ⓐ	ⓑ	ⓒ	ⓓ		90.	ⓐ	ⓑ	ⓒ	ⓓ		145.	ⓐ	ⓑ	ⓒ	ⓓ
36.	ⓐ	ⓑ	ⓒ	ⓓ		91.	ⓐ	ⓑ	ⓒ	ⓓ		146.	ⓐ	ⓑ	ⓒ	ⓓ
37.	ⓐ	ⓑ	ⓒ	ⓓ		92.	ⓐ	ⓑ	ⓒ	ⓓ		147.	ⓐ	ⓑ	ⓒ	ⓓ
38.	ⓐ	ⓑ	ⓒ	ⓓ		93.	ⓐ	ⓑ	ⓒ	ⓓ		148.	ⓐ	ⓑ	ⓒ	ⓓ
39.	ⓐ	ⓑ	ⓒ	ⓓ		94.	ⓐ	ⓑ	ⓒ	ⓓ		149.	ⓐ	ⓑ	ⓒ	ⓓ
40.	ⓐ	ⓑ	ⓒ	ⓓ		95.	ⓐ	ⓑ	ⓒ	ⓓ		150.	ⓐ	ⓑ	ⓒ	ⓓ
41.	ⓐ	ⓑ	ⓒ	ⓓ		96.	_____					151.	ⓐ	ⓑ	ⓒ	ⓓ
42.	ⓐ	ⓑ	ⓒ	ⓓ		97.	ⓐ	ⓑ	ⓒ	ⓓ		152.	ⓐ	ⓑ	ⓒ	ⓓ
43.	ⓐ	ⓑ	ⓒ	ⓓ		98.	ⓐ	ⓑ	ⓒ	ⓓ		153.	ⓐ	ⓑ	ⓒ	ⓓ
44.	ⓐ	ⓑ	ⓒ	ⓓ		99.	ⓐ	ⓑ	ⓒ	ⓓ		154.	ⓐ	ⓑ	ⓒ	ⓓ
45.	ⓐ	ⓑ	ⓒ	ⓓ		100.	ⓐ	ⓑ	ⓒ	ⓓ		155.	ⓐ	ⓑ	ⓒ	ⓓ
46.	ⓐ	ⓑ	ⓒ	ⓓ		101.	ⓐ	ⓑ	ⓒ	ⓓ		156.	ⓐ	ⓑ	ⓒ	ⓓ
47.	ⓐ	ⓑ	ⓒ	ⓓ		102.	ⓐ	ⓑ	ⓒ	ⓓ		157.	ⓐ	ⓑ	ⓒ	ⓓ
48.	ⓐ	ⓑ	ⓒ	ⓓ		103.	ⓐ	ⓑ	ⓒ	ⓓ		158.	ⓐ	ⓑ	ⓒ	ⓓ
49.	_____					104.	ⓐ	ⓑ	ⓒ	ⓓ		159.	ⓐ	ⓑ	ⓒ	ⓓ
50.	ⓐ	ⓑ	ⓒ	ⓓ		105.	ⓐ	ⓑ	ⓒ	ⓓ		160.	ⓐ	ⓑ	ⓒ	ⓓ
51.	ⓐ	ⓑ	ⓒ	ⓓ		106.	ⓐ	ⓑ	ⓒ	ⓓ		161.	ⓐ	ⓑ	ⓒ	ⓓ
52.	_____					107.	ⓐ	ⓑ	ⓒ	ⓓ		162.	ⓐ	ⓑ	ⓒ	ⓓ
53.	_____					108.	ⓐ	ⓑ	ⓒ	ⓓ		153.	ⓐ	ⓑ	ⓒ	ⓓ
54.	_____					109.	ⓐ	ⓑ	ⓒ	ⓓ		164.	ⓐ	ⓑ	ⓒ	ⓓ
55.	ⓐ	ⓑ	ⓒ	ⓓ		110.	ⓐ	ⓑ	ⓒ	ⓓ		165.	ⓐ	ⓑ	ⓒ	ⓓ

Questions

1. A male client being treated on a mental health unit becomes angry and belligerent toward the nursing staff after an argument with a family member. If the client's anger escalates after alternative measures fail and he refuses a p.r.n. sedative medication, the nurse has which of the following legal options?
   a. The client has the right to refuse the medication and the nurse must respect the client's rights.
   b. The nurse can administer the p.r.n sedative to protect the safety of the patient and others.
   c. The nurse must contact a probate court judge and get permission to administer the medication.
   d. The nurse should contact the hospital's attorney related to the client's right to refuse treatment.

2. The nurse is assessing the growth and development of a toddler. The nurse knows that according to Erik Erickson's stages of psychosocial development, the toddler is in the stage of
   a. autonomy versus shame and doubt.
   b. industry versus inferiority.
   c. initiative versus guilt.
   d. trust versus mistrust.

3. The nurse is coordinating care for a woman who is 6-hours postpartum for hemorrhagic shock. The nurse knows that signs/symptoms of hemorrhagic shock include
   a. cool, clammy skin.
   b. lochiarubra.
   c. urinary output < 30 mL per hour.
   d. uterine cramping.

4. The nurse is caring for a client with hypertension. On the illustration, identify the area where the nurse will place the stethoscope to best auscultate the pulmonic valve.

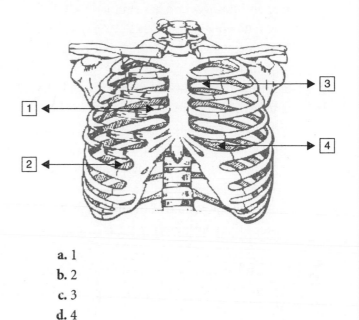

   a. 1
   b. 2
   c. 3
   d. 4

5. The nurse manager of a mental health unit is reviewing a chart entry made by a staff member. The entry reads: "I feel unloved; appears confused and restless." Which of the following statements best describes why this nursing documentation is incorrect?
   a. The nurse who made this chart entry failed to document that the client made the quote.
   b. The nurse who made this chart entry failed to explore/interpret the client's feelings of being "unloved."
   c. The nurse who made this chart entry failed to indicate the importance of the client's statement(s).
   d. The nurse who made this chart entry failed to accurately describe the evidence of confusion and restlessness.

6. A mother brings a 12-month-old child to the pediatrician's office for an influenza vaccination. Before administering the immunization, the nurse notes the child is acting fussy, is warm and flushed, and has rhinorrhea. Which of the following is the nurse's priority action?

a. assessing the child for additional symptoms of febrile illness

b. advising the mother that since the child has a fever the immunization will need to be given at a later date

c. providing the child with cool fluids to reduce the fever and applying an anesthetic cream to the injection site

d. notifying the pediatrician and obtaining an order for an antipyretic

7. An infant has been transferred from the NICU to the pediatric unit following surgery to correct a heart defect. Which of the following tasks are within the scope of practice for a licensed practical nurse (LPN)? Select all that apply.

1. administering oral medications
2. administering IV morphine
3. administering blood products
4. discharge teaching
5. morning hygiene
6. recording the input and output

a. 1, 2, 3, 4, 5

b. 2, 4, 5, 6

c. 1, 5, 6

d. 3, 6

8. The nurse is preparing to take a blood pressure (BP) reading on a client. Which of the following actions demonstrate appropriate technique? Select all that apply.

1. centering the bladder of the BP cuff over the brachial artery
2. inflating the BP cuff 30 mm Hg above the reading where the brachial pulse disappears
3. utilizing a BP cuff that is 80% of arm circumference
4. quickly releasing the bulb valve so the pressure drops more than 10 mm Hg per second
5. wrapping the BP cuff so that the lower border is 8 cm above the antecubital space

a. 1, 2, 4, 5

b. 1, 2, 3

c. 2, 3, 5

d. 1, 4

9. A 5-year-old female child is brought to the local clinic by her parents to prepare for school entry. The parents report the child has not had any vaccinations since she was 5 months old. To determine the current best practices for scheduling missed vaccinations the nurse will complete which of the following?

a. check the CDC (Centers for Disease Control and Prevention) website

b. consult the child's primary physician

c. contact the local pharmacist

d. read the vaccines manufacturers' inserts

10. The nurse determines the body mass index (BMI) for a 7-year-old boy to be 15.5. According to the chart, this places the child at which percentile?

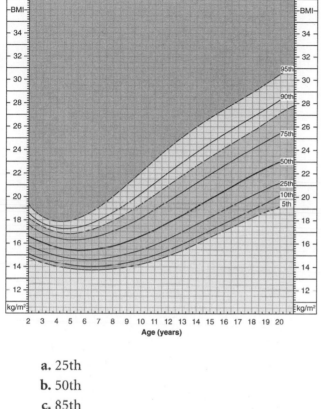

Age (years)

    a. 25th
    b. 50th
    c. 85th
    d. 95th

11. A client has just lost his job. He says he's worried that he won't be able to afford his mortgage. The nurse knows that mild levels of anxiety can cause which of the following?
    a. fixation
    b. motivation for growth
    c. panic attack
    d. sense of impending doom

12. The unit director of a medical surgical floor asks a graduate LPN, "Based on the HIPAA [Health Insurance Portability and Accountability Act] regulations, what client information is protected and should not be disclosed?" The graduate correctly states which of the following? Select all that apply.
    1. client's address
    2. client's computer password
    3. client's date of birth
    4. client's insurance information
    5. client's occupation
    6. client's medical condition
    7. client's social security number
    a. 1, 3, 4, 6, 7
    b. 1, 3, 5, 7
    c. 2, 4, 6
    d. 3, 5, 7

13. The nurse is caring for a client on a medical surgical unit diagnosed with pneumonia. The nurse should instruct the nursing assistant also caring for the client to report which of the information immediately?
    a. dry mouth/mucous membranes
    b. nonproductive cough
    c. pink-colored skin
    d. restlessness

14. The nurse is assisting in the coordination of care for a woman in labor. The chart documents the fetal station as +1. The nurse knows that this means that the fetal head is one centimeter
    a. above the ischeal spines.
    b. above the cervix.
    c. below the ischeal spines.
    d. below the cervix.

15. The nurse is participating in the care of a client with laryngeal cancer. The client has undergone a laryngectomy and is receiving head and neck radiation. The nurse correctly identifies which of the following as adverse side effects of external radiation? Select all that apply.

    1. dysgeusia

    2. cystitis

    3. leukopenia

    4. stomatitis

    5. thrombocytopenia

    6. xerostomia

a. 1, 2, 3, 4, 5, 6

b. 3, 4, 5, 6

c. 1, 4, 5

d. 1, 3

16. A pregnant woman is admitted into the hospital due to preterm labor. She tells the nurse that she is going to go home right now because she cannot stand being in the hospital another minute. Which of the following should the nurse do first?

a. call security to stop the client

b. notify the registered nurse

c. place the client in restraints

d. tell the client she cannot leave

17. The nurse is caring for a female client with an enlarged spleen. Identify the quadrant of the abdomen where the nurse would find the enlarged spleen.

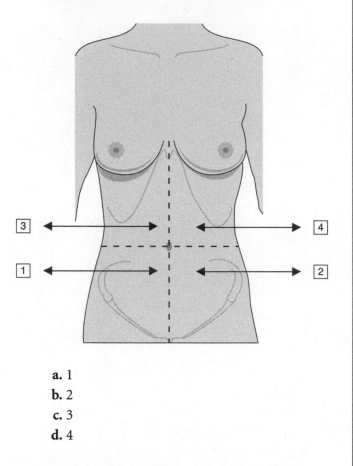

a. 1

b. 2

c. 3

d. 4

18. The nurse is caring for a client who is ordered to receive Neupogen (filgrastim) subcutaneously after receiving cytotoxic chemotherapy. The physician has ordered 5 mcg/kg, the client weighs 150 pounds, and Neupogen is supplied in a vial of 300 mcg/mL. How many mLs of Neupogen will the client receive?

a. 5.5

b. 1.05

c. 1.13

d. 0.95

19. A nurse is participating in a staff development program on illicit drug overdose. The nurse recognizes additional teaching is not needed when a staff member states that clients with suspected cocaine overdose are at risk for
a. cardiac arrest.
b. lethargy.
c. psychosis.
d. respiratory arrest.

20. The nurse is supervising a newly hired nursing assistant. The nursing assistant (NA) is providing oral care to an unconscious client. Which of the following actions made by the NA would indicate that the NA requires further instructions from the LPN?
a. ensuring the client remains in the lateral position for 30 minutes after oral care
b. placing a towel under the client's chin prior to completing oral care
c. positioning the client in an upright position while providing oral care
d. placing the client in the lateral position with the head turned to the side during oral care

21. The nurse is caring for multiple clients on a restraint-free nursing unit. She is concerned about preventing falls. Which of the following tasks would be inappropriate for the nurse to delegate to the nursing assistant?
a. assessing the safety needs of the client
b. ensuring the client's bed is in the lowest position
c. monitoring client's behavior for potential falls
d. placing frequently used objects within the client's reach

22. The nurse is documenting a 10-year-old girl's BMI on the chart shown here and finds that the girl's BMI is in the 25th percentile. The nurse knows that according to the BMI chart, this child is

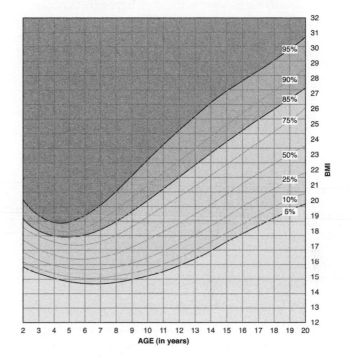

a. underweight.
b. of healthy weight.
c. overweight.
d. obese.

23. The home care nurse is visiting a 72-year-old male client diagnosed with Alzheimer's disease. During the visit, the nurse observes bruising on the client's forearms and legs. The client is also more withdrawn than normal. The client is unable to communicate effectively because of his disease progression. The nurse suspects elder abuse. What is the nurse's responsibility in this situation?

a. continue to monitor the situation during subsequent visits

b. do nothing because the nurse has no proof of actual abuse

c. report the suspicion to the local agency on aging within 24 hours

d. try and convince the client to report the situation

24. The LPN is caring for six clients in a nursing home with the help of a nursing assistant. Which of the following tasks can the LPN delegate to the nursing assistant?

a. assisting a client to the bathroom and documenting the appearance of the stool

b. auscultating and documenting the client's breath sounds in the medical record

c. notifying the physician of a change in the client's heart rate

d. taking the verbal report for a client being transferred to the nursing home

25. The nurse is attempting to establish a therapeutic relationship with a client. The nurse knows that the process can be facilitated by

a. commenting on the client's behavior.

b. demonstrating a nonjudgmental attitude.

c. giving the client advice.

d. sympathizing with the client.

26. The nurse is assessing the growth and development of a preschooler. The nurse knows that, according to Erik Erickson's stages of psychosocial development, the preschooler is in the stage of

a. autonomy versus shame and doubt.

b. industry versus inferiority.

c. initiative versus guilt.

d. trust versus mistrust.

27. The nurse is providing care to a 10-year-old who is blind. Which communication technique is the most appropriate?

a. announce presence when entering the room

b. face the child when explaining procedures

c. speak in a loud, slow manner

d. quietly leave the room

28. The nurse is working with a pregnant client who states that she is worried because she does not have enough money to buy food. The nurse identifies _____ as a resource that provides supplemental nutrition and nutritional education for low-income pregnant women, as well as postpartum women and children under the age of 5 who are at nutritional risk.

29. A client brings a newborn infant to the emergency room and states that she does not want to keep the infant. The nurse knows that the client is not required to provide her name according to which of the following laws/regulations?

a. HIPAA

b. Medicaid

c. Safe Haven

d. WIC

30. The nurse is participating in the care of a client admitted to the medical-surgical unit with a diagnosis of acute pyelonephritis. The nurse understands that which of the following nursing interventions is a priority while caring for this client?

 a. administering a sitz bath twice per day to the client

 b. ensuring the client drinks cranberry juice to acidify the urine

 c. increasing the client's fluid intake to 3 liters per day

 d. inserting a urinary catheter to measure urine output accurately

31. The nurse is assisting in the provision of education on nutrition for a group of pregnant women. The nurse knows that further teaching is indicated when one of the participants states that she will avoid/eliminate which of the following from her diet?

 a. alcohol

 b. eggs

 c. sushi

 d. unpasteurized juice

32. The nurse is caring for a client in end-stage renal failure. The client is ordered to receive 100 units/kg of Procrit (epoetin alfa) subcutaneously. The client weighs 70 kg and the Procrit is supplied in a 20,000 unit/mL vial. How many mLs of Procrit will the nurse administer?

 a. 0.7

 b. 0.9

 c. 0.35

 d. 1.1

33. The nurse is caring for a client with a stage-II pressure ulcer to the left heel. It is most appropriate for the nurse to consult which of the following disciplines in the care of this client?

 a. nutritional support and orthotics

 b. occupational therapy and infectious disease

 c. plastic surgery and cardiology

 d. physical and respiratory therapy

34. A nurse is collecting data on a client admitted to the inpatient mental health unit. The client is complaining of sleep disturbances, feelings of helplessness, and a loss of appetite. The nurse recognizes these symptoms to be indicative of:

 a. anxiety

 b. bipolar disorder

 c. delusional disorder

 d. depression

35. The nurse is caring for a client with a spinal cord injury. The client is a tetraplegic. On the illustration, identify the area of the spinal cord where the injury most likely occurred.

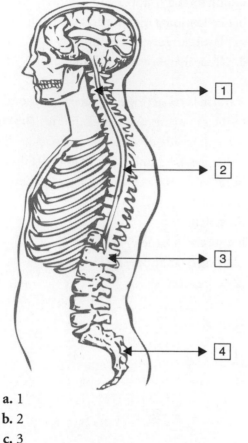

    a. 1
    b. 2
    c. 3
    d. 4

36. The nurse is caring for a client with end-stage renal failure. Which of the following statements by the client best demonstrates an understanding of an advance directive?

    a. "A living will allows my decisions for healthcare to be known if I can't speak for myself."

    b. "I will rely on my primary physician to do whatever is best for me; I don't need a living will."

    c. "Once I decide on an advance directive, I can never change my mind."

    d. "An attorney will allow my son to use my funds to pay for my healthcare costs, if I can't do so."

37. The nurse is caring for a female client 3 days post a total right hip replacement. The client asks the nurse why she must go to a rehabilitation facility. Which of the following is the best response by the nurse?

    a. "The physician wants you to go to the rehabilitation center until you are able to care for yourself."

    b. "The rehabilitation staff can evaluate your progress and make sure that you exercise without risking injury."

    c. "The rehabilitation staff can provide you with better care than the hospital staff."

    d. "You'll need help with your daily activities for quite some time."

38. A nurse is changing the dressing on a postpartum woman whose cesarean incision line dehisced due to an abscess. When performing the dressing change, the nurse should utilize which of the following types of techniques/maneuvers?

    a. aseptic
    b. fundal massage
    c. Leopold's
    d. sterile

39. The nurse knows that which of the following decreases an infant's risk for Sudden Infant Death Syndrome (SIDS)? Select all that apply.

    1. supine sleep position
    2. use of a pacifier
    3. prone sleep position
    4. stuffed animals in the crib
    a. 1 and 2
    b. 1 and 4
    c. 2 and 3
    d. 3 and 4

40. The nurse is assisting in the care of a pregnant client. The nurse obtains a blood pressure reading of 160/98 and +1 protein in the client's urine. There is no evidence/documentation of seizure activity. The nurse identifies that the client is exhibiting symptoms of
   a. eclampsia.
   b. pre-eclampsia.
   c. preterm labor.
   d. uterine atony.

41. The nurse is assisting at a disaster setup following a flood. The nurse recognizes that the most common problem she will likely see in the clients at the shelter is which of the following?
   a. exacerbation of existing medical problems
   b. traumatic injuries
   c. thirst
   d. stress

42. The nurse is caring for a client who has developed a stage-III pressure ulcer due to prolonged immobility. The nurse understands that even though the client has been turned and repositioned every 2 hours per protocol since hospitalization, pressure ulcers may develop from
   a. inadequate massaging of the affected area.
   b. inadequate protein intake.
   c. inadequate vitamin D intake.
   d. low calcium levels.

43. The nurse is reinforcing cord care education for a young mother of a neonate. Which of the following actions would the nurse expect the mother to complete during this procedure? Select all that apply.
   1. Apply antibiotic ointment to the cord once daily.
   2. Clean the length of the cord with alcohol several times daily.
   3. Keep the diaper below the cord.
   4. Only sponge bathe the infant until the cord falls off.
   5. Tug the cord gently as the cord dries.
   6. Wash the cord with mild soap and water.
   a. 1, 2, 4, 6
   b. 3, 4, 5, 6
   c. 1, 2, 3
   d. 2, 3, 4

44. The nurse is caring for an infant with severe diarrhea. Which of the following room assignments is best for this infant?
   a. a private room
   b. a room in close proximity to the nurse's station
   c. a room with another infant who has diarrhea
   d. a room with a child who has a broken arm

45. The nurse is assisting in the discharge of a new mother and her newborn. The nurse states that the newborn should travel home from the hospital in the
   a. front seat in a rear-facing infant car seat.
   b. front seat in a forward-facing infant car seat.
   c. back seat in a rear-facing infant car seat.
   d. back seat in a forward-facing infant car seat.

46. The nurse is collecting data on a client admitted with post-traumatic stress disorder (PTSD). Which symptoms would the nurse expect to find during the data collection?

1. continuous discussion of the event
2. difficulty concentrating
3. difficulty maintaining close relationships
4. repetitive behaviors

a. 1 and 2
b. 2 and 3
c. 3 and 4
d. 1 and 4

47. The nurse is participating in the care of a 17-year-old male client with a comminuted fracture of the right distal tibia that required surgery. The client returned from surgery four hours ago. The nurse recognizes which of the following as the highest priority when reassessing and documenting postoperative circulation of the casted leg?

a. minimal pain upon movement of the extremity
b. no drainage observed on the cast
c. normal VS (vital signs)
d. satisfactory neurovascular functioning

48. The nurse is reinforcing nutritional education to a pregnant client. The nurse should state that the client should consume no more than how many milligrams of caffeine per day?

a. 100
b. 200
c. 300
d. 400

49. The nurse will determine a child's body surface area by using a/an _____.

50. The nurse is participating in the care of a client experiencing an anaphylactic reaction related to a bee sting. The physician orders epinephrine 1:1000 aqueous solution 0.5 subcutaneously. The nurse has obtained a prefilled syringe of 1:1000 1mg/mL. How many mLs will the nurse administer?

a. 1
b. 2
c. 0.25
d. 0.5

51. The home health nurse is completing a follow-up visit for a client diagnosed with AIDS. Which behavior, if observed by the nurse, indicates a need for further instruction?

a. The client uses the same razor as other family members.
b. The client uses the same dishes and utensils as the rest of the family.
c. The client uses the same bathroom as the rest of the family.
d. The client cooks meals regularly for the family.

52. The nurse is administering digoxin (Lanoxin) elixir to a toddler diagnosed with heart failure. Prior to administering this medication, the nurse must check the toddler's

_____.

53. A client who is diagnosed with mycoplasma pneumonia needs to leave the nursing unit for an X-ray. The client should wear a/an

_____ _____.

54. The nurse has completed caring for a client who is in a contact isolation room. Prior to leaving the room the nurse needs to remove her protective gear/wear. Place the following steps in chronological order as to how the protective wear should be removed. Use all the options.

1. remove eye shield
2. remove gloves
3. remove gown
4. remove mask
5. wash hands for no less than 15 seconds

55. A client brings her 9-month-old who has a high fever to the ER. Which action should the nurse suggest to the mother to promote the infant's comfort during the exam?
a. continue holding the infant
b. not offering the infant the pacifier
c. giving the infant to the nurse
d. placing the infant on the exam table

56. The nurse is caring for a client diagnosed with an embolic stroke secondary to atrial fibrillation. On the illustration, identify the heart chamber that is most likely the source of the fragmented clot responsible for the client's stroke.

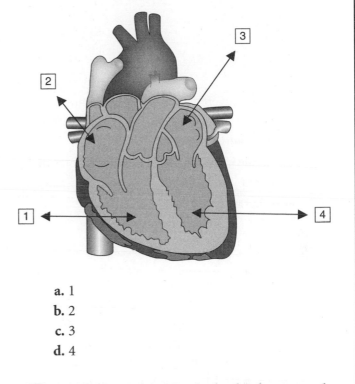

a. 1
b. 2
c. 3
d. 4

57. A nurse is participating in the development of a plan of care for an infant with a diaper rash (dermatitis). Which intervention should be included in the plan of care?
a. barrier cream application
b. cleansing only after bowel movements
c. not exposing diaper area to the air
d. yeast ointment application

58. The nurse is participating in the care of a client who states that she is the Tooth Fairy. The nurse should
a. agree that the client is the Tooth Fairy.
b. ask the client when she first realized this.
c. tell the client she is not the Tooth Fairy.
d. tell the client the Tooth Fairy is not real.

59. The nurse is assessing a pregnant client for pitting edema. When the nurse presses her index and middle fingers against the client's shin there is a 6 mm pit and it takes 11 seconds for the pit to rebound. The nurse should document the edema as

a. +1.

b. +2.

c. +3.

d. +4.

60. A client delivered an infant with Dandy-Walker syndrome. The nurse overhears the client tell a friend that the infant is "perfectly fine." The nurse knows that this statement indicates that the client is in which stage of grief?

a. acceptance

b. anger

c. bargaining

d. denial

61. The nurse is assisting in an educational program for pregnant women. In a discussion of newborns, the nurse indicates that the neonate's first stool, the _____ stool, will be tarry and dark green or black in appearance.

62. The nurse is participating in the care of a client 30 hours after major surgery. The nurse notes the client has a temperature of 100.8 degrees F. The nurse understands that the most likely cause of this temperature elevation is which of the following?

a. atelectasis

b. bladder infection

c. dehydration

d. wound infection

63. The nurse is reinforcing discharge plans for a 3-year-old admitted with croup. The nurse knows that further education is needed when the mother states that she will

a. place the child in a steamy bathroom when symptomatic.

b. increase the child's fluid intake.

c. take the child out in the cool air when symptomatic.

d. use a dehumidifier in the child's bedroom.

64. The nurse is working in a long-term nursing facility and smells smoke in the hallway. Upon entering a client's room, she notes the client is sitting up in a chair and the blankets on the client's bed are on fire. The nurse takes immediate action. Place the nurse's actions in proper chronological order. Use all the options.

_____

1. confine the fire
2. extinguish the fire
3. rescue the client
4. trigger the alarm

65. The nurse is caring for a client on an oncology unit. The client is diagnosed with thrombocytopenia. Which of the following actions is the best way for the nurse to protect the client?

a. document accurate fluid intake and output on the medical record

b. instruct the client to use a wheelchair as often as possible

c. restrict the client's visitations from family and friends

d. utilize the smallest needle when administering injections

66. The nurse is reviewing the proper procedure for transferring a client from the bed to a wheelchair. Which of the following actions should the nurse take during this client transfer?
   a. help the client dangle his legs on the side of the bed
   b. stand behind the client during the transfer
   c. place the chair facing toward the foot of the bed during the transfer
   d. position the head of the bed in the flat position

67. The nurse is participating in the care of a client who is scheduled for an elective cardioversion. Before the procedure is attempted, the nurse correctly holds which of the following medications?
   a. Coumadin (warfarin)
   b. digoxin (Lanoxin)
   c. heparin (liposodium)
   d. Valium (diazepam)

68. The nurse is performing wound care utilizing surgical asepsis. Which of the following practices does NOT ensure the surgical asepsis technique?
   a. considering a $1-1\frac{1}{2}$ inch edge around the sterile field contaminated
   b. holding sterile objects above the waistline
   c. opening the outermost flap of a sterile package away from the body
   d. pouring solution onto a sterile field cloth

69. The nurse is reinforcing teaching with the parents of a child with an ileostomy. The nurse explains that which part of the intestines, as labeled here, is brought to the abdominal surface to create the stoma?

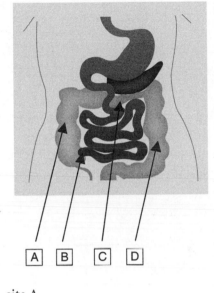

   a. site A
   b. site B
   c. site C
   d. site D

70. A male client is admitted to a medical-surgical unit with a diagnosis of Guillain-Barré syndrome. On the fourth day of hospitalization, the client's compromised muscle strength worsens, and he is unable to stand. The client is also experiencing difficulty swallowing and talking. The nurse recognizes the client is at the greatest risk for developing
   a. aspiration pneumonia.
   b. bladder distension.
   c. decubitus ulcers.
   d. hypertensive crisis.

71. The nurse performs a Weber's test on a client who presents to the community clinic complaining of difficulty hearing. The nurse correctly identifies which of the following locations to place the tuning fork to perform the Weber's test?

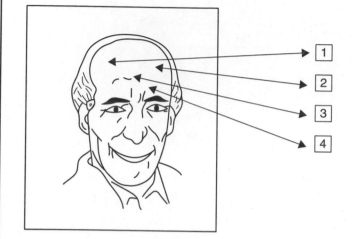

  a. 1
  b. 2
  c. 3
  d. 4

72. The nurse is assisting in the screening of a client for domestic violence. The nurse should utilize which of the following screening tools?
  a. SKIN
  b. BSE
  c. HITS
  d. PSA test

73. The nurse is reinforcing teaching to a woman experiencing morning sickness. The nurse knows additional education is needed when the client states that she will eat/drink
  a. water with each meal.
  b. dry crackers in the morning.
  c. small frequent meals.
  d. bland foods.

74. The nurse is reinforcing proper latching on technique with a new mother who is breast feeding her neonate. During correct latch-on, where on the breast should the neonate's lips be located?
  a. breast tissue
  b. areola
  c. base of nipple
  d. tip of nipple

75. The nurse is assisting in the care of a 2-day-old Hispanic newborn. While changing the diaper, the nurse notes the following.

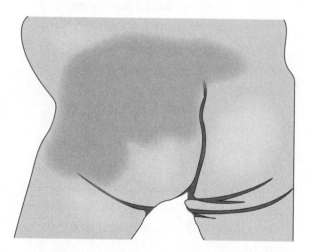

The nurse should document
  a. abuse.
  b. milia.
  c. Mongolian spots.
  d. Montgomery tubercles.

76. The nurse is ambulating with a female client in the hallway of the nursing unit. Suddenly, the client complains of dizziness and feeling faint. What is the nurse's priority action in this situation?
  a. ease the client to a sitting position
  b. instruct the client to put her head between her legs
  c. instruct the client to walk faster
  d. quickly go and obtain help from the nursing staff

77. The nurse needs to assess and palpate a client's dorsalis pedis pulse. Identify the area where the nurse places her fingers to palpate the pedal pulse.

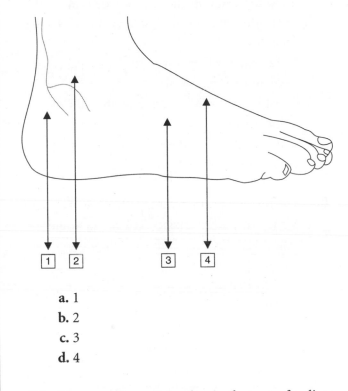

a. 1

b. 2

c. 3

d. 4

78. The nurse is participating in the care of a client who must have a routine screening for colorectal cancer. The nurse needs to obtain a fecal sample for occult blood testing. Which of the foods should the nurse instruct the client to avoid 48 to 72 hours before the test and throughout the collection period? Select all that apply.

1. cantaloupe
2. fish
3. high-fiber foods
4. peas
5. tomatoes
6. turnips

a. 1, 4, 5, 6

b. 2, 3, 4, 5

c. 1, 2, 6

d. 1, 4

79. The nurse is caring for a client two days after abdominal surgery. The nurse encourages the client to take deep breaths and cough. The client refuses, stating, "It hurts too much when I cough, I just can't do it." What is the nurse's best response?

a. "After you complete the deep breathing and coughing activities, I will give you pain medication."

b. "Put a pillow over your incision to support your incision, then breathe deeply and cough."

c. "Okay, we can wait for four hours and then you must try again to cough and breathe deeply."

d. "You have to cough and breathe deeply or you may develop pneumonia."

80. The nurse is participating in the care of a male client diagnosed with liver failure. Daily measurements of his abdominal girth are ordered. Identify where the nurse will place the tape measure when obtaining this measurement.

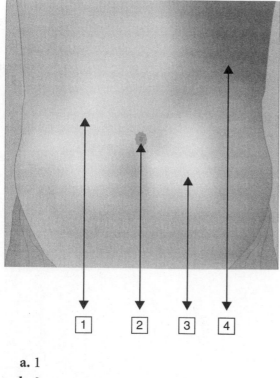

a. 1
b. 2
c. 3
d. 4

81. A newborn is ordered an IM injection of vitamin K. Where should the nurse administer the injection?
a. deltoid muscle
b. dorsogluteal muscle
c. vastuslateralis muscle
d. rectus femoris muscle

82. The nurse is participating in the care of a client who is to undergo a PTCA (percutaneous transluminal coronary angioplasty). The physician has prescribed 81 mg of aspirin daily. The nurse understands the best explanation for this medication therapy in this situation is which of the following?
a. Aspirin can help relieve any chest pain the client may experience.
b. Aspirin can aid in decreasing blood clot formation.
c. Aspirin helps to lower blood pressure.
d. Aspirin tends to dilate the coronary arteries.

83. The nurse is participating in the care of a client with anticipatory anxiety. The nurse would expect the client to exhibit which of the following?
a. fear constantly present
b. fear of what will happen next
c. mistrust and suspicion of others
d. sense of impending doom

84. The nurse is measuring the length of an abscessed, open area of a cesarean incision. To document the wound's length, the nurse converts the 2.2 inches length obtained to _____ cm.

85. A client arrives at a physician's office to schedule a series of tests/examinations to rule out prostate cancer. The nurse recognizes that to avoid false test results, the nurse should schedule which of the following diagnostic tests prior to the client receiving a rectal examination?
a. KUB (kidneys, ureters, bladder X-ray)
b. PSA (prostatic-specific antigen)
c. MRI (magnetic resonance imaging)
d. needle biopsy of the prostate gland

86. The nurse is assigned to care for an adolescent client who overdosed on acetylsalicylic acid (aspirin). The nurse expects to care for a client with which of the following? Select all that apply.

    1. jaundice

    2. oliguria

    3. abdominal pain

    4. tinnitus

  a. 1 and 3

  b. 2 and 4

  c. 1 and 4

  d. 2 and 3

87. The nurse is caring for a client diagnosed with pernicious anemia. Which of the following assessments can the nurse expect to find?

  a. increased appetite

  b. decreased platelet count

  c. ecchymosis on the client's trunk

  d. neuropathy of the lower extremities

88. The nurse is participating in the care of a pediatric client with appendicitis. The nurse knows that pain from appendicitis occurs in which part of the abdomen?

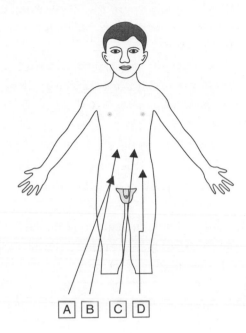

  a. part A

  b. part B

  c. part C

  d. part D

89. The nurse is assisting in a community education program on the prevention of lead poisoning. The nurse should include information that screening tests for lead poisoning include

  a. blood levels of lead.

  b. bone X-rays for lead therapy.

  c. chelation therapy.

  d. kidney function test.

90. The nurse is participating in the care of a client admitted to a nursing home for bladder training after a traumatic brain injury. The client tells the nurse, "I'm not drinking a lot so I can stay dry longer." Which of the following responses by the nurse is most appropriate in this situation?
   a. Encourage the client to keep restricting fluids because this is evidence of client cooperation.
   b. Encourage the client to restrict fluids as it will help obtain the client's goals of care.
   c. Discourage the client from restricting fluids because this may contribute to a fluid imbalance.
   d. Tell the client adequate fluid intake is necessary to help prevent the development of constipation.

91. The nurse is participating in the care of a client with an ostomy. Which of the following suggestions if made by the nurse to the client will be most helpful to control urine leakage when the apparatus is being changed?
   a. "Lean over the toilet when changing the appliance."
   b. "Place a gloved finger in the stoma when changing the appliance."
   c. "When changing the appliance, insert a tampon into the stoma."
   d. "When you change the appliance, pinch the stoma with two fingers."

92. The nurse is caring for a client with hepatitis A. The nurse is aware that which of the following factors can cause hepatitis A?
   a. blood transfusions with infected blood
   b. contact with infected blood
   c. eating contaminated shellfish
   d. sexual contact with an infected person

93. The nurse is assisting in the development of the plan of care for a client experiencing a manic episode. The plan of care should include assessment for which of the following?
   a. decreased self-esteem
   b. increased sleeping
   c. increased appetite
   d. weight loss

94. The nurse is participating in the care of a client who is diagnosed with a panic disorder. The nurse is aware that which of the following physical signs and symptoms may be experienced during a panic attack? Select all that apply.
   1. bradycardia
   2. delayed speech
   3. diarrhea
   4. dizziness
   5. shortness of breath
   6. sweating
   a. 1, 2, 4, 5, 6
   b. 1, 3, 4, 5
   c. 3, 4, 5, 6
   d. 1, 2

95. The nurse is preparing to give betamethasone (Celestone) to a pregnant client in preterm labor. The nurse knows that this medication should be administered by which of the following routes?
   a. oral
   b. intramuscular
   c. intravenous
   d. sublingual

96. To decrease the risk for urinary tract infections, young girls should be instructed to wipe the perianal area from _____ to _____ after bowel movements.

97. The nurse is assisting in the care of a pregnant mother with gestational diabetes. The nurse knows that the risk factors for gestational diabetes include which of the following?
a. alcohol consumption
b. maternal age < 35
c. obesity
d. preterm labor

98. The nurse is assisting in the care of a laboring client when the client's water breaks. The fluid is yellow in color. The nurse suspects
a. placental abruption.
b. fetal distress.
c. infection.
d. normal amniotic fluid.

99. The nurse is participating in the care of a newly admitted client to a chemical dependency unit. The client's drug screen is positive for cocaine. The nurse should monitor the client for which of the following?
a. bradycardia
b. elevated blood glucose levels
c. ECG changes/dysrhythmias
d. depressed respirations

100. The nurse is participating in the care of a female client newly diagnosed with multiple sclerosis (MS). The nurse recognizes which of the following is true?
a. MS can be related to mosquito bites.
b. MS can occur in persons who have had the chicken pox.
c. MS is considered an autoimmune condition/disease.
d. MS often follows a streptococcal infection.

101. The nurse is contributing to the plan of care for a client with hemophilia A. Which of the following would NOT be included?
a. administration of frozen factor VIII
b. administration of platelets
c. immobilization of impacted joints
d. implementation of bleeding precautions

102. The nurse is caring for a client participating in a chemical dependency day program. The nurse suspects the client has been smoking marijuana prior to arrival. The nurse understands which of the following signs are associated with recent marijuana usage? Select all that apply.
1. increased sexual drive
2. inflamed eyes
3. pinpoint pupils
4. restlessness
5. shivering
6. tachycardia
a. 1, 2, 3, 5
b. 3, 4, 5, 6
c. 1, 3, 4
d. 2, 6

103. The nurse is caring for a client who is receiving 5,000 units of heparin sodium subcutaneously. The nurse will review which of the following laboratory results prior to administering the injection?
a. CBC
b. Hb
c. PT
d. PTT

104. The nurse is reinforcing teaching with the parents of a child diagnosed with phenylketonuria (PKU) on the prevention of central nervous system damage from toxic levels of phenylalanine. The nurse realizes additional teaching is needed when the parents state that the child will need to avoid which of the following?

a. aspartame

b. fish

c. ice cream

d. jelly

105. The nurse is assisting in the development of the plan of care for a child with esophageal atresia. The plan of care should include which of the following?

a. aspiration precautions

b. increased fluids

c. supine position

d. tracheal suction

106. The nurse is participating in the care of a male client diagnosed with post-traumatic stress disorder (PTSD). Which of the following is the most therapeutic and beneficial intervention for a client diagnosed with PTSD?

a. administering antianxiety medications per order

b. encouraging the client to express his feelings openly

c. monitoring the client's physical symptoms

d. observing the client's interactions with family and friends

107. The nurse is participating in the care of a client who is to undergo a cardiac catheterization and arteriogram. The client is very anxious about the procedure. Which of the following nursing actions can best help to decrease the client's anxiety?

a. avoiding speaking to the client about the catheterization until the client is relaxed and ready

b. explaining that the procedure is generally very helpful for most clients

c. listening to the client's feelings about the hospitalization and about his or her condition

d. reinforcing to the client how coronary artery disease is commonly treated

108. The nurse is caring for a client admitted to the hospital with a myocardial infarction. On the second day of admission, the client begins to have hand tremors and experiences anxiety and a shaky feeling. Which assessment data should the nurse assist in collecting?

a. alcohol consumption

b. blood pressure

c. hemoglobin A1c

d. medication

109. The nurse is participating in the care of a client with cerebral palsy. The chart states that the client has athetosis. The nurse expects the client to exhibit

a. diminished reflexes.

b. involuntary writhing motions.

c. rigidity.

d. uncoordinated muscle movement.

110. The nurse is assisting in the plan of care for a client with dissociative amnesia disorder. The nurse plans care for a client with
   a. alternating periods of euphoria and depression.
   b. gradual loss of mental abilities.
   c. loss of personal memories.
   d. loss of personal reality.

111. The nurse is caring for an 80-year-old female client on a cardiac telemetry unit. The client becomes scared/startled when an ECG lead becomes loose and the monitor alarm sounds. Which of the following nursing actions will best relieve the client's anxiety?
   a. administering the client's prescribed tranquilizer
   b. describing the client's current cardiac rhythm
   c. showing the client a tracing of her heart rhythm
   d. telling the client why the monitor alarm sounded

112. The nurse is documenting the weight of a 5-year-old boy in kilograms. The weight obtained on the scale is 43 pounds. The nurse should document the boy's weight as which of the following?
   a. 15.3 kg
   b. 19.5 kg
   c. 43.0 kg
   d. 45.0 kg

113. The nurse is participating in the care for a client whose cultural background is different from her own. Which of the following nursing actions are most appropriate when interacting with this client? Select all that apply.
   1. Consider that nonverbal cues (e.g., eye contact) may have a different meaning in different cultures.
   2. Explain the nurse's beliefs to the client so the client will understand the differences.
   3. Inquire whether there are any cultural or religious requirements that should be considered in the client's care.
   4. Respect the client's cultural beliefs.
   5. Understand that all cultures experience pain in the same way.
   a. 1, 2, 3, 4, 5
   b. 1, 3, 4
   c. 2, 4, 5
   d. 1, 2

114. The nurse is participating in the care of a client who is terminally ill. The client states, "I know I'm going to die today." Which of the following is the best response by the nurse?
   a. "Don't worry, you aren't going to die."
   b. "Oh, no, you're doing quite well considering your condition."
   c. "We have equipment to monitor you and your problems."
   d. "Why do you think you're going to die today?"

115. The nurse is participating in the care of a female client who has undergone a modified radical mastectomy. The client is ordered to receive Nolvadex (tamoxifen) 10 mg po twice daily for the treatment of her estrogen-sensitive breast cancer. There are 20 mg in each tablet. How many tablets should the nurse administer to the client?

a. 1
b. 2
c. 0.5
d. 0.75

116. The nurse is administering eardrops to a 4-year-old girl. The nurse should gently pull the pinna

a. down and back.
b. down and out.
c. up and back.
d. up and out.

117. The nurse is caring for a male client with chronic renal failure. The client receives hemodialysis and is also a diabetic. The client asks whether it is acceptable to take his insulin shot prior to hemodialysis. The nurse recognizes that which of the following statements is true and should be included in the nurse's reply to the client?

a. The hemodialysis treatment will destroy the injected insulin.
b. The hemodialysis treatment actually stimulates insulin production.
c. Insulin levels are not reduced by the hemodialysis treatment.
d. Insulin will enhance the effects of the hemodialysis treatment.

118. The nurse is caring for a client diagnosed with renal failure who requires daily weighings. The nurse directs the nursing assistant (NA) to obtain the client's weight. Which of the following instructions is most important for the nurse to tell the nursing assistant in order for the NA to obtain accurate data?

a. Ask the client about his/her normal/predisease weight.
b. Obtain the client's weight utilizing a bedside scale.
c. Tell the client to remove his/her footwear prior to weighing.
d. Weigh the client at the same time each day and on the same scale.

119. The nurse receives a report from the lab that a client's lithium level is 1.9 mEq/L. Which of the following might the client be experiencing?

a. agitation
b. drooling
c. headache
d. tremors

120. The nurse is caring for a 30-year-old client diagnosed with ulcerative colitis. The client is experiencing bowel incontinence. Which of the following nursing interventions is most appropriate when managing this client?

a. answering the client's call bell promptly
b. assisting the client to the bathroom often
c. ensuring the client has on a disposable brief at all times
d. keeping a portable commode at the bedside

121. The nurse is assisting a newborn infant and recognizes which of the following should be reported to the physician?

a. bulging posterior fontanel
b. cephalohematoma
c. molding of infant's head
d. open posterior fontanel

122. The nurse is caring for a client who is ordered colostomy irrigations. Which of the following positions is best to place the client in when performing the irrigations?
a. kneeling over the bathtub
b. lying on the left side
c. sitting on the toilet
d. standing over the sink

123. The nurse is caring for a client complaining of pain (7/10 on the pain scale). The nurse will administer the client's prescribed Demerol (meperidine hydrochloride). The client is ordered 50 mg I.M. and the medication is supplied in a 100 mg/mL ampule. What amount should the nurse administer?
a. 0.2 mL
b. 0.5 mL
c. 1.0 mL
d. 2.0 mL

124. The nurse is administering amoxicillin to a child. The order reads 500 mg of amoxicillin q 4 hours. On hand is amoxicillin 125 mg/tsp. How many teaspoons should the nurse administer?
a. 0.25 teaspoons
b. 2 teaspoons
c. 3 teaspoons
d. 4 teaspoons

125. The nurse is caring for a client with a tracheostomy. The client requires suctioning. The nurse understands that while withdrawing the suction catheter from the client's tracheostomy tube, which of the following techniques is correct?
a. Pinch and pull the catheter.
b. Remove the catheter slowly.
c. Thrust the catheter up and down.
d. Twist and rotate the catheter.

126. The nurse is participating in the care of a client diagnosed with exacerbation of MS (multiple sclerosis). The nurse is planning the care of the client. Which of the following is the best approach when assisting the client with ADLs (activities of daily living)?
a. Eliminate any activities the client cannot complete alone.
b. Have the client complete ADLs in 30-minute increments.
c. Have the client rest between activities.
d. Perform all the client's ADLs.

127. The nurse is administering Proventil as a metered dose inhalation. The nurse should administer the medication
a. as the child is exhaling.
b. as the child is inhaling.
c. just prior to the child inhaling.
d. just prior to the child exhaling.

128. The nurse is assisting in planning care for an elderly client prescribed Ativan. The plan should include which of the following?
a. assess for hypertension
b. assess for megaloblastic anemia
c. implement fall precautions
d. implement suicide precautions

129. The nurse is assisting in the determination of a neonate's Apgar score. Which of the following will be included in the assessment?
1. heart rate
2. respiratory effort
3. sucking reflex
4. urinary output
a. 1 and 2
b. 2 and 3
c. 1 and 4
d. 2 and 4

130. A client is admitted to a medical-surgical unit for the treatment of gout. The nurse recognizes the client is at risk of developing urinary stones. The client is ordered to consume 3,000 mL of fluid daily. The most appropriate time for the client to consume the majority of fluid is

    a. before bedtime.

    b. early evening.

    c. in the morning.

    d. midafternoon.

131. The nurse is participating in the care of a client who is exhibiting signs of hypovolemic shock. Which of the following client findings is most likely to be present?

    a. decreased heart rate

    b. decreased respiratory rate

    c. decreased urinary output

    d. elevated systolic and lowered diastolic BP

132. The nurse is participating in the care of a client diagnosed with tetraplegia. The client is experiencing severe muscle spasms. The client is ordered baclofen (Lioresal), 5 mg orally three times daily. The nurse understands the principal indication for baclofen is

    a. acute, painful musculoskeletal conditions.

    b. muscle spasms from spinal cord lesions.

    c. skeletal muscle hyperactivity secondary to cerebral palsy.

    d. spasticity related to cerebrovascular accident.

133. The nurse is assisting in the plan of care for a 1-year-old child with hydrocephalus. The nurse includes which assessment in the plan of care?

    a. sunken fontanel

    b. increased activity

    c. widening suture lines

    d. decreased blood pressure

134. The nurse is caring for a client with a cystostomy for urine drainage. Identify the area on the following image where the nurse should check for cystostomy placement.

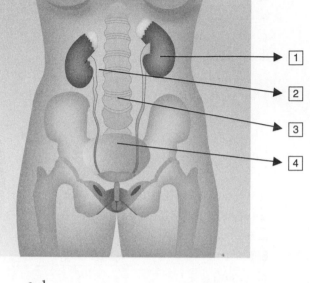

    a. 1

    b. 2

    c. 3

    d. 4

135. The nurse is participating in the care of a client diagnosed with left-sided heart failure. While caring for the client, the nurse should monitor which of the following on a daily basis?

    a. appetite

    b. peripheral edema

    c. pupil response

    d. weight

136. A client has end-stage metastatic lung cancer and is taking IV morphine for pain management. The nurse notices that the client has needed an increasingly stronger dosage of the medication to control her pain. The nurse recognizes that the client is experiencing which of the following?

    a. dependency

    b. substance abuse

    c. tolerance

    d. withdrawal

137. The nurse is preparing to administer prosta-glandin E to a laboring client. The purpose of the medication is to
  a. increase uterine contractions.
  b. treat eclampsia.
  c. relieve labor pain.
  d. ripen the cervix.

138. The nurse is participating in the care of a client who is to receive a sodium phosphate enema for constipation. The proper administration of the enema includes which of the following steps? Select all that apply.
  1. Allow gravity to instill the enema solution.
  2. Assist the client to the Sims' position.
  3. Chill the solution in the refrigerator for 10 minutes.
  4. Encourage the client to retain the solution for 5 to 15 minutes.
  5. Insert the tip of the container 0.5" into the rectum.
  6. Wash hands per protocol and put on gloves.
  a. 1, 2, 4, 5, 6
  b. 3, 4, 5, 6
  c. 2, 4, 6
  d. 1, 3

139. A client is prescribed the benzodiazepine Xanax. The nurse knows that this medication is used to treat which of the following?
  a. alcohol abuse
  b. anxiety
  c. delirium
  d. depression

140. A client is on continuous jevity tube feedings via NG tube at 30 cc per hour. What should the nurse ask the nursing assistant to do prior to placing the client in a supine position during a bed bath?
  a. check the feeding tube's placement
  b. decrease the rate to 20 cc per hour
  c. disconnect the feeding tube
  d. place the feeding on hold

141. The nursing care plan includes off-loading pressure from the client's heels. To implement this intervention, the nurse should
  a. place a pillow under the client's heels.
  b. place the client in heel lifts.
  c. position the client in a supine position.
  d. position the client in a high-Fowler's position.

142. The nurse observes two nursing assistants talking about a client's test results in a cafeteria where visitors can easily hear the conversation. The nurse explains to the assistants that this is a _____ violation.

143. The nurse is reinforcing teaching about antacid therapy for a client who has been diagnosed with a gastric ulcer and who is preparing for discharge. The nurse's follow-up teaching should include which of the following instructions?
  a. "Avoid taking magnesium-containing antacids if you develop a heart problem."
  b. "Be sure to take the antacids with meals."
  c. "Continue to take antacids even if your symptoms go away."
  d. "You can take the antacids with your other medications."

144. The nurse is contributing to a staff development program on ostomy care and management. The nurse realizes that additional teaching is not needed when a staff member states that the ostomy pouch should be emptied when it is:

a. $\frac{1}{4}$ full

b. $\frac{1}{3}$ full

c. $\frac{3}{4}$ full

d. $\frac{7}{8}$ full

145. The nurse is participating in the care of a male client with severe burn injuries. The client had skin grafting completed five hours ago. What nursing care measures/activities are appropriate at the graft site the day of the grafting?

a. change the graft site dressing twice daily

b. elevate the recipient site

c. help the client complete range-of-motion activities

d. leave the graft site open to air

146. The nurse is making a follow-up phone call to a client who was placed on Coumadin therapy and was discharged the previous day. The nurse knows that the client understands the teaching when the client states that his INR should be between

a. 0 and 1.

b. 1 and 2.

c. 2 and 3.

d. 3 and 4.

147. Which of the following healthcare team members would the nurse expect to have been consulted for a client having difficulties with fine motor movement?

a. occupational therapist

b. physical therapist

c. recreational therapist

d. speech therapist

148. The nurse is assisting in the well-child assessment of a 13-year-old girl. When the child bends over and touches her toes, the nurse observes the following:

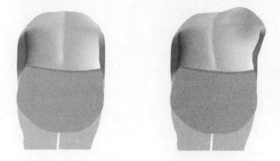

The nurse knows that this client should be evaluated for

a. dowager's hump.

b. kyphosis.

c. scoliosis.

d. uneven leg length.

149. The nurse is assisting in the development of a plan of care for a client in left-sided heart failure. One of the interventions is assessment for signs and symptoms of this condition including which of the following?

a. hepatomegaly

b. jugular vein distension

c. orthopnea

d. right upper quadrant pain

150. The nurse is participating in the plan of care for a client who was diagnosed with a delusional disorder with erotomania subtype. The nurse assists in planning care for a client with an irrational belief of which of the following?

a. bodily nonfunctionality or disfigurement

b. conspiracy against him or her

c. love from person with higher social status

d. unfaithfulness from his or her significant other

151. The nurse is participating in the care of a client diagnosed with diabetes insipidus. The nurse should anticipate administering which of the following medications?
   a. furosemide (Lasix)
   b. insulin
   c. potassium chloride
   d. vasopressin (Pitressin)

152. The nurse is reinforcing discharge teaching for a client with an abdominal wound. What dietary instruction should be included to promote wound healing?
   a. decreased dietary fats
   b. 2 gm sodium diet
   c. increased protein
   d. increased carbohydrates

153. The nurse is assisting in the care of a client with a diabetic leg ulcer. The physician has planned to debride the wound in the morning, but the client, who is alert and oriented, tells the nurse that she changed her mind and does not want to have the debridement. The nurse should tell the client which of the following?
   a. "Everything will be okay."
   b. "I will let your physician know."
   c. "The debridement will be tomorrow."
   d. "This is a common procedure."

154. The nurse is assisting in the delivery of a staff educational program on organ donation. The nurse recognizes additional teaching is needed when a staff member states which of the following are contraindications to organ donation?
   a. age more than 65
   b. trauma
   c. malignancy
   d. communicable disease

155. The nurse is caring for a client with MRSA in his wound. Prior to entering the room to perform the dressing change, the nurse should do which of the following? Select all that apply.
   1. wash hands
   2. put on a gown
   3. put on gloves
   4. put on a mask
   a. 1, 2, 3
   b. 2, 3, 4
   c. 1, 2, 4
   d. 1, 3, 4

156. The nurse is assisting in gathering data about a client with schizophrenia. The client states that he is "hearing voices." Which is the appropriate action by the nurse?
   a. Ask what the voices are saying.
   b. Move the client to a room by the nursing station.
   c. Contact the registered nurse.
   d. Tell the client no one else is in the room.

157. A client admitted with a seizure disorder is being discharged on a daily dose of Depakene (valproic acid). The nurse reviewing the discharge instructions with the client realizes that the best time for the client to take the medication is before
   a. breakfast.
   b. lunch.
   c. dinner.
   d. bed.

158. The nurse is caring for clients on a medical-surgical unit. When the nurse is making rounds on her assigned clients, she finds a client who is not breathing and has no pulse. After the nurse calls for help, what should she do next?
   a. administer five chest compressions
   b. give/administer two rescue breaths
   c. retrieve the code/emergency cart
   d. quickly defibrillate the client

159. The nurse is caring for a client whose right lower extremity is shiny and hairless. The nurse is unable to palpate a pedal pulse. The nurse should
  a. assess the pulse with a Doppler.
  b. check the capillary refill time.
  c. contact the physician.
  d. elevate the extremity.

160. The nurse is participating in the care of a client diagnosed with TB (tuberculosis). The client is prescribed rifampin (Rafadin). The client complains of gastrointestinal side effects after taking the medication. Which of the following is the nurse's best course of action?
  a. administer the medication at bedtime
  b. administer the medication with food
  c. administer the medication with an antacid
  d. encourage the client to drink more water

161. The nurse is caring for a client with Alzheimer's disease who has a history of wandering. Which is the most appropriate nursing intervention to promote this client's safety?
  a. bed/chair alarm
  b. lowboy bed
  c. vest restraints
  d. wrist restraints

162. A client is receiving systemic radiation. The nurse knows that this client is at risk for which of the following?
    1. dysgeusia
    2. leukopenia
    3. thrombocytopenia
    4. xerostomia
  a. 1 and 2
  b. 1 and 3
  c. 2 and 3
  d. 2 and 4

163. A client is unable to reposition herself in the bed. To prevent a hospital-acquired pressure ulcer from occurring, the nurse should be sure that the client is repositioned every
  a. 30 minutes.
  b. 1–2 hours.
  c. 2–3 hours.
  d. shift.

164. The nurse is entering the room of a client on droplet precautions to take the client's blood pressure. The nurse should put on which of the following protective equipment?
    1. gloves
    2. goggles
    3. gown
    4. mask
  a. 1, 2, 3
  b. 2, 3, 4
  c. 1, 2, 4
  d. 1, 3, 4

165. The nurse working in an OB-GYN practice knows that risk factors for breast cancer include all the following EXCEPT
  a. first pregnancy over the age of 35.
  b. first period after age 12.
  c. high breast-density.
  d. postmenopausal weight gain.

Answers

1. b. The nurse can administer medications to a client against his or her will when the circumstances indicate a potential for danger to the client or others. The nurse must provide objective and complete documentation describing the circumstances and the failure of alternative measures. Choice **a** is incorrect. Under most circumstances the nurse should respect the client's right to refuse treatment; however, when the circumstances indicate a potential for danger to the client or others, the client's rights are waived. Choice **c** is incorrect. The nurse does not need to receive permission from a judge to administer the p.r.n. medication. Choice **d** is incorrect. The hospital's attorney does not need to be notified.
Category: Safe and Effective Care Environment: Coordination of Care
Subcategory: Mental Health

2. a. Autonomy versus shame and doubt occurs during the toddler years. Choice **b** is incorrect. Industry versus inferiority occurs during the school-age years. Choice **c** is incorrect. Initiative versus guilt occurs during the preschool years. Choice **d** is incorrect. Trust versus mistrust occurs during the infant period.
Category: Health Promotion and Maintenance
Subcategory: Pediatrics: Growth and Development

3. c. Urinary output of less than 30 mL/hour is indicative of inadequate organ perfusion and oxygenation and can be an indicator of hemorrhagic shock. Choice **a** is incorrect. Cool, clammy skin is a symptom of shock. Choice **b** is incorrect. Lochiarubra is the term for the normal, red, bloody vaginal discharge that occurs in the first week after delivery. Choice **d** is incorrect. Uterine cramping in the early postpartum period assists with involution of the uterus and is not indicative of hemorrhagic shock.
Category: Safe and Effective Care Environment: Coordinated Care
Subcategory: Maternal Infant: Postpartum

4. c. The pulmonic valve is best heard at the second intercostal space, at the left sternal border.
Category: Physiological Integrity: Physiological Adaptation
Subcategory: Cardiovascular Disorders

5. d. The nurse should report what was observed, as words such as "confused" and "restless" may not mean the same to all heathcare providers. Reporting what was actually observed is a much more accurate and objective method for documenting behavior. Accurate documentation is essential as the nurse's notes become a part of the client's permanent record and can be used as evidence in a court of law. Choice **a** is incorrect. The question doesn't reference whether the nurse documented who was speaking, so this answer is inappropriate. Choice **b** is incorrect. The nurse should report what is objectively observed, and avoid attempting to interpret the client's feelings. Choice **c** is incorrect. The nurse should not attempt to judge the importance of a client's statements in his or her documentation/charting.
Category: Safe and Effective Care Environment: Coordination of Care
Subcategory: Mental Health

6. a. The nurse should assess the child for additional information about the illness. Acute febrile illness is generally considered a contraindication for the administration of immunizing agents because side effects are additive to existing illness and the symptoms of the two will be confused. Choice **b** is incorrect. Advising the mother that the appointment may need to be rescheduled is appropriate; however, the priority action is to further assess the child. Choice **c** is incorrect. Providing the child with fluids may be appropriate, but the priority action is to further assess the child. Choice **d** is incorrect. Notifying the physician and obtaining an order for an antipyretic may be appropriate, but the priority action is to further assess the child.

Category: Safe and Effective Care Environment: Coordination of Care

Subcategory: Pediatrics

7. c. The RN's scope of practice includes all components of the nursing process. Only aspects of care implementation may be completed by the LPN. The exact skills that may be completed by the LPN vary by state and institution. In general, LPNs can administer oral medications (1), perform hygiene (5), and record intake and output (6). LPNs can also obtain vital signs. The LPN can reinforce discharge teaching after it is initially imitated by the RN (4). Administering IV medications and blood products is completed by the RN.

Category: Safe and Effective Care Environment: Coordination of Care

Subcategory: Pediatrics

8. b. The nurse recognizes that to obtain an accurate BP reading, the following must be done: she should center the bladder of the BP cuff over the brachial artery; the BP cuff should be inflated 30 mm Hg above the reading where the brachial pulse disappears to ensure an accurate assessment of the systolic BP; and the bladder of the BP cuff must be 80% of the arm circumference. The following should also be done: the bulb valve should be released slowly so pressure drops about 2–3 mm Hg per second, not 10 mm Hg, because inaccurate measurements may occur if the deflation rate is faster; the nurse should wrap the BP cuff so that the lower border of the cuff is 2 cm, not 8 cm, above the antecubital space, with the bladder centered over the brachial artery.

Category: Physiological Integrity: Reduction of Risk

Subcategory: Miscellaneous

9. a. The CDC is the federal body that is responsible for vaccination recommendations for children as well as adults. The CDC publishes current vaccination catch-up schedules that are readily available on their website. Choice **b** is incorrect. The lack of vaccinations is a strong indicator that the child probably does not have a primary care physician. Choice **c** is incorrect. The pharmacist would probably also review the CDC guidelines that are equally available to the nurse. Choice **d** is incorrect. Reading the manufacturer's inserts for multiple vaccinations can be confusing and time consuming, and has a high potential to lead to errors.

Category: Safe and Effective Care Environment: Coordination of Care

Subcategory: Pediatrics

10. b. If a 7-year-old boy has a BMI of 15.5, the BMI is in the 50th percentile. Choice **a** is incorrect. If the child's BMI was in the 25th percentile, the BMI would be 13.5. Choice **c** is incorrect. If the child's BMI was in the 85th percentile, the BMI would be 17.5. Choice **d** is incorrect. If the child's BMI was in the 95th percentile, the BMI would be 19.
Category: Health Promotion and Maintenance
Subcategory: Pediatrics: Growth and Development

11. b. Mild levels of anxiety can provide motivation for growth. Choice **a** is incorrect. Fixation, the inability to focus on anything but a fear or worry, occurs in moderate to severe levels of anxiety. Choice **c** is incorrect. Panic attacks occur in panic disorders. Choice **d** is incorrect. A sense of impending doom occurs with panic levels of anxiety.
Category: Psychosocial Integrity
Subcategory: Mental Health: Anxiety

12. a. The HIPAA regulations were enacted by the federal government to protect clients' health information. HIPAA maintains confidentiality and regulates those who can access client records. Protected information includes: client's address, date of birth, insurance information, medical condition, social security number, phone number, past and present medical history, or future plans for treatment. HIPAA regulations do not include the client's occupation or passwords, although computer passwords should always be kept secure. Choices **b**, **c**, and **d** are incorrect. See the rationale for choice **a** for explanation.
Category: Safe and Effective Care Environment: Coordination of Care
Subcategory: Medical Surgical: Miscellaneous

13. d. The nurse should be made aware if the client develops restlessness. Restlessness is a sign of hypoxia and a client diagnosed with pneumonia should be assessed for it. It is within the scope of practice of a nursing assistant to report restlessness to the nurse. Choice **a** is incorrect. Dry mouth/mucous membranes are a common finding in a client diagnosed with pneumonia because these clients are often mouth-breathers. Choice **b** is incorrect. A nonproductive cough would require further assessment, but is not as crucial as assessing restlessness. Choice **c** is incorrect. Pink-colored skin is a normal assessment finding and would not need to be reported immediately.
Category: Safe and Effective Care Environment: Coordination of Care
Subcategory: Medical Surgical: Respiratory Disorders

14. c. When the fetal head is 1 cm below the ischeal spines, the fetal station is documented as +1. Choice **a** is incorrect. When the fetal head is 1 cm above the ischeal spines, it is documented as −1. Choices **b** and **d** are incorrect. Fetal station refers to the location of the fetal head in relation to the ischeal spines, not the cervix.
Category: Safe and Effective Care Environment: Coordinated Care
Subcategory: Maternal Infant: Intrapartum

15. c. External radiation of the head and neck often causes dysgeusia, stomatitis, and thrombocytopenia. Cystitis may occur more commonly after radiation of the GI system; leukopenia and xerostomia may be experienced after systemic radiation.
Category: Physiological Integrity: Reduction of Risk
Subcategory: Oncology Disorders

16. b. The licensed practical nurse should notify the registered nurse. If the client is insistent on leaving the facility, the registered nurse should be notified so that he or she can ask the client to sign the appropriate documents relating to leaving against medical advice. Choice **a** is incorrect. Clients have the right to refuse healthcare and/or leave the facility at any time. Security is not legally able to prevent them from leaving. Choice **c** is incorrect. Placing the client in restraints is considered false imprisonment. Choice **d** is incorrect. Clients have the right to refuse healthcare and/or leave the facility at any time.
Category: Safe and Effective Care Environment: Coordinated Care
Subcategory: Maternal Infant: Antepartum Complications

17. d. The spleen is located in the left upper abdominal quadrant, posterior to the stomach.
Category: Physiological Integrity: Physiological Adaptation
Subcategory: Miscellaneous

18. c. The calculation is as follows:
$$\frac{150 \text{ lb}}{2.2 \text{ kg}} = 68 \text{ kg}$$
$$68 \text{ kg} \times 5 \text{ mcg} = 340 \text{ mcg/kg}$$
$$\frac{300}{1} = \frac{340}{x}$$
$$\frac{340}{300} = 1.13$$
$$x = 1.13 \text{ mL}$$
Category: Physiological Integrity: Pharmacology
Subcategory: Oncology Disorders

19. a. The client with a cocaine overdose is at risk for cardiac arrhythmias, which can lead to cardiac arrest. Choice **b** is incorrect. Lethargy is associated with an overdose of sedatives. Choice **c** is incorrect. Psychosis is associated with an overdose of hallucinogens. Choice **d** is incorrect. Respiratory arrest is associated with an overdose of narcotics.
Category: Physiological Integrity: Reduction of Risk
Subcategory: Mental Health: Chemical Dependency

20. c. The client should not be placed in this position. The unconscious client will be unable to maintain an upright position without falling or tilting to the side. The LPN would need to intervene and provide further education/instructions on the proper procedure for providing oral care to a comatose client. Choice **a** is incorrect. This is correct procedure and prevents pooling of secretions and aspiration of fluids. Choice **b** is incorrect. This is correct procedure and keeps the area dry and clean. Choice **d** is incorrect. This is correct procedure and will protect the client from aspirating.
Category: Safe and Effective Care Environment: Coordination of Care
Subcategory: Medical Surgical: Neurological Disorders

21. a. The LPN is responsible for assessing the safety needs of the client and should not delegate this task to the nursing assistant. Choice **b** is incorrect. The bed should be in the lowest position to prevent injuries resulting from falling. It is appropriate for the LPN to delegate this task. Choice **c** is incorrect. Monitoring the behavior of the client is within the scope of practice for a nursing assistant and can be delegated by the LPN. Assessment of the behavior and problem solving is the role of the LPN. Choice **d** is incorrect. Frequently used items should be placed within the client's reach to prevent falls. It is appropriate for the LPN to delegate this task.
Category: Safe and Effective Care Environment: Coordination of Care
Subcategory: Medical Surgical: Miscellaneous

22. b. A girl whose BMI is between the 5th and 85th percentile is considered to be at a healthy weight. Choice **a** is incorrect. A girl whose BMI is less than the 5th percentile is considered underweight. Choice **c** is incorrect. A girl whose BMI is between the 85th and 95th percentile is considered to be overweight. Choice **d** is incorrect. A girl whose BMI is greater than the 95th percentile is considered to be obese.
Category: Health Promotion and Maintenance
Subcategory: Pediatrics: Growth and Development

23. c. The nurse must report the suspicion of abuse to the local agency on aging within 24 hours of the visit. Choices **a** and **b** are incorrect. These options go against the nurse's legal and professional obligation, which is to report suspected abuse when it occurs. Choice **d** is incorrect. The client's disease process prevents him from reporting the problem to the appropriate agency.
Category: Safe and Effective Care Environment: Coordination of Care
Subcategory: Medical Surgical: Neurological Disorders

24. a. The nurse can safely delegate activities of daily living such as assisting the client to the bathroom to the nursing assistant. Choice **b** is incorrect. Auscultating and documenting breath sounds is the responsibility of the nurse. Choice **c** is incorrect. Notifying the physician is the responsibility of the nurse. Choice **d** is incorrect. Taking the verbal report is a responsibility that must be performed by the nurse.
Category: Safe and Effective Care Environment: Coordination of Care
Subcategory: Medical Surgical: Musculoskeletal Disorders

25. b. To facilitate the establishment of a therapeutic relationship, the nurse should demonstrate a nonjudgmental attitude. Choice **a** is incorrect. Commenting on the client's behavior demonstrates a judgmental attitude, which can hinder the establishment of a therapeutic relationship. Choice **c** is incorrect. The nurse should not give the client advice as a part of a therapeutic relationship. Choice **d** is incorrect. The nurse should emphathize with the client versus sympathize.
Category: Psychosocial Integrity
Subcategory: Mental Health: Therapeutic Relationship

26. c. Initiative versus guilt occurs during the preschool years, according to Erickson's stages of psychosocial development. Choice **a** is incorrect. Autonomy versus shame and doubt occurs during the toddler years, according to Erickson's stages of psychosocial development. Choice **b** is incorrect. Industry versus inferiority occurs during the school-age years, according to Erickson's stages of psychosocial development. Choice **d** is incorrect. Trust versus mistrust is the stage for infants, according to Erickson's stages of psychosocial development.
Category: Health Promotion and Maintenance
Subcategory: Mental Health: Psychosocial Development

27. a. The nurse should announce his or her presence when entering the room. Choice **b** is incorrect. Facing the child when explaining procedures is important if the child has a hearing deficit, but will not facilitate communication with a child who is blind. Choice **c** is incorrect. Speaking in a loud, slow manner will not facilitate communication with a child who is blind. Choice **d** is incorrect. If the nurse quietly leaves the room, the child who is blind might not realize that the nurse is gone.
Category: Physiological Integrity: Basic Care and Comfort
Subcategory: Pediatrics: Sensory Deficits

28. The correct answer is *Women, Infants and Children (WIC)*
Women, Infants and Children (WIC) is a federally funded resource that provides supplemental nutrition, health referrals, and nutritional education for pregnant women, postpartum women, and children under the age of 5 who are at nutritional risk.
Category: Safe and Effective Care Environment: Coordinated Care
Subcategory: Maternal Infant: Antepartum

29. c. According to Safe Haven laws/regulations, a mother can leave her newborn at any hospital emergency room if she does not want to keep the infant and does not have to provide her name. Choice **a** is incorrect. HIPAA regulations address the protection of clients' healthcare information. Choice **b** is incorrect. Medicaid regulations address eligibility and payment for care provided. Choice **d** is incorrect. WIC regulations address eligibility of pregnant women, postpartum women, and children under the age of 5 for nutritional supplementation, healthcare referrals, and nutritional education.
Category: Safe and Effective Care Environment: Coordinated Care
Subcategory: Maternal Infant: Antepartum

30. c. The nurse is aware that pyelonephritis is a sudden inflammation of the interstitial tissue and renal pelvis of one or both kidneys. Infecting bacteria are normal intestinal and fecal flora that grow readily in the urine. Pyelonephritis may result from procedures that involve the use of instruments or from hematogenic infection. The highest-priority nursing intervention is for the nurse to increase the client's fluid intake to 3 liters daily. The increased fluid consumption helps empty the bladder of contaminated urine and prevents stone formation. Choice **a** is incorrect. Administering a sitz bath to the client would increase the likelihood of fecal contamination. Choice **b** is incorrect. Encouraging the client to drink cranberry juice to acidify urine is helpful but is not the most important/priority nursing intervention. Choice **d** is incorrect. Inserting an indwelling urinary catheter could cause further contamination.

Category: Physiological Integrity: Reduction of Risk

Subcategory: Renal Disorders

31. b. While consuming raw and undercooked eggs places the woman at risk for salmonella poisoning, completely cooking the eggs eliminates this risk. Fully cooked eggs are an appropriate source of protein for pregnant clients. Choice **a** is incorrect. Current guidelines call for the elimination of alcohol from the pregnant woman's diet due to the risk of fetal abnormalities. Choice **c** is incorrect. Sushi contains illness-producing parasites and should be avoided by pregnant women. Choice **d** is incorrect. Unpasteurized juices contain contaminants that can harm the fetus. (Most juices sold in supermarkets are pasteurized and therefore are safe for consumption by the pregnant woman.)

Category: Safe and Effective Care Environment: Safety and Infection Control

Subcategory: Maternal Infant: Antepartum

32. c. The calculation is as follows:

$$70 \text{ kg} \times 100 \text{ mg} = 7,000 \text{ mg/kg}$$

$$\frac{20,000 \text{ units}}{1 \text{ mL}} = \frac{7,000 \text{ units}}{x}$$

$$\frac{7,000}{20,000} = 0.35$$

$$x = 0.35$$

Category: Physiological Integrity: Pharmacology

Subcategory: Renal Disorders

33. a. Nutritional support should be consulted to evaluate the client's caloric needs for wound healing. Orthotics should also be consulted for specialized footwear designed to keep pressure off the client's left heel. Choice **b** is incorrect. Occupational therapy may be utilized to assist with activities of daily living, but consulting infectious disease isn't necessary unless the client has a coexisting infection. Choice **c** is incorrect. A plastic surgery consult may be necessary if debridement or grafting is needed, but nothing indicates that a cardiology consult is needed. Choice **d** is incorrect. Physical therapy is necessary to help the client get to optimal functioning; however, a respiratory consult is not necessary because the scenario does not state that the client has any coexisting respiratory problem/disease.

Category: Safe and Effective Care Environment: Coordination of Care

Subcategory: Medical Surgical: Integumentary Disorders

34. d. Symptoms of depression include sleep disturbances, feelings of helplessness, and loss of appetite. Choice **a** is incorrect. Symptoms of anxiety include unrealistic worry, diaphoresis, sleep disturbances, inability to concentrate, pacing, and forgetfulness. Choice **b** is incorrect. Symptoms of bipolar disorder include periods of euphoria alternating with periods of depression. Choice **c** is incorrect. Symptoms of delusional disorders include false beliefs (delusions) and hallucinations.
Category: Psychosocial Integrity
Subcategory: Mental Health: Depression

35. a. Tetraplegia, also known as quadriplegia, is paralysis caused by illness or injury that results in the partial or total loss of use of limbs and torso. The loss is usually both sensory and motor, which means that both sensation and control are lost. It is caused by damage to the brain or the spinal cord at the C1–C7 level, that is, spinal cord injuries secondary to an injury to the cervical spine.
Category: Physiological Integrity: Physiological Adaptation
Subcategory: Neurological Disorders

36. a. An advance directive is a document written in the form of a living will. It expresses the client's wishes about healthcare, providing direction for the physician if the client becomes terminally ill and can't express his or her wishes. Choice **b** is incorrect. The client should not depend on the physician to make his or her healthcare decisions. Choice **c** is incorrect. A client can change his or her mind about advance directives at any time. Choice **d** is incorrect. An attorney allows the client to designate another person to make healthcare decisions for the client in case the client becomes too ill to make his or her own decisions.
Category: Safe, effective care environment: Coordination of Care
Subcategory: Medical Surgical: Advanced Directives

37. b. This choice explains the role of the rehabilitation staff. Choice **a** is incorrect. This response does not explain the specific ways the the rehabilitation center will aid the client's recovery. Choice **c** is incorrect. This response is judgmental about the care the hospital staff may provide and doesn't adequately explain the role of a rehabilitation center in the client's recovery. Choice **d** is incorrect. This response doesn't provide adequate information about the role of rehabilitation or the client's future needs and makes an assumption about the amount of time the client may need help.
Category: Safe and Effective Care Environment: Coordination of Care
Subcategory: Medical Surgical: Musculoskeletal Disorders

38. a. The LPM should utilize aseptic technique, which is used to prevent the spread of unwanted organisms. Choice **b** is incorrect. Fundal massage is utilized in the early postpartum period when the uterine tone is noted to be soft or boggy. Choice **c** is incorrect. Leopold's maneuvers are utilized to determine the fetal lie during the late prenatal period and early stages of labor. Choice **d** is incorrect. Sterile technique is utilized to prevent infection of surgical wounds. The patient already has an abscess—resulting from an infection—therefore the nurse needs to apply aseptic technique in caring for the abscess.
Category: Safe and Effective Care Environment: Safety and Infection Control
Subcategory: Maternal Infant: Post partum

39. a. Both the use of a pacifier (2) and placing the infant in a supine (on the back) sleep position (1) decrease the risk for SIDS. Choice **b** is incorrect. Placing the infant in a supine (on the back) sleep position (1) decreases the risk for SIDS but sleeping with stuffed animals in the crib (4) increases the infant's risk for SIDS. Choice **c** is incorrect. While use of a pacifier (2) decreases the risk of SIDS, placing the infant in a prone (on the stomach) sleep position (3) increases the risk for SIDS. Choice **d** is incorrect. Placing the infant in a prone (on the stomach) sleep position (3) and keeping stuffed animals in the crib (4) both increase the infant's risk for SIDS.
Category: Safe and Effective Care Environment: Safety and Infection Control
Subcategory: Maternal Infant: Neonate

40. b. Elevated blood pressure and protein in the urine are symptoms of pre-eclampsia in the pregnant client. Choice **a** is incorrect. For the client to be exhibiting signs of eclampsia, there would need to be evidence/documentation of seizure activity. Choice **c** is incorrect. Symptoms of preterm labor include abdominal cramping and contractions accompanied by cervical dilation. Choice **d** is incorrect. Uterine atony is a condition that occurs in the postpartum period. Symptoms include a boggy uterus.
Category: Safe and Effective Care Environment: Safety and Infection Control
Subcategory: Maternal Infant: Antepartum

41. d. Stress is the most common problem seen/encountered in a disaster situation. Choices **a**, **b**, and **c** are incorrect. Even though clients may report experiencing exacerbation of existing medical problems, traumatic injuries, and thirst, the most common problem seen in a disaster shelter is stress.
Category: Safe and Effective Care Environment: Safety and Infection Control
Subcategory: Mental Health Disorders

42. b. Clients on bed rest suffer from a lack of movement and a negative nitrogen balance; inadequate intake of protein, the amino acids of which contain nitrogen, impairs wound healing. Even if the client is repositioned every two hours, protein pressure sores may develop and may not heal as desired. Choice **a** is incorrect. A pressure ulcer should never be massaged. Choice **c** is incorrect. Inadequate vitamin D intake is not a factor in poor healing for this client. Choice **d** is incorrect. A low calcium level is not a factor in poor healing for this client.
Category: Physiological Integrity: Reduction of Risk
Subcategory: Integumentary Disorders

43. d. The length of the cord should be cleaned with alcohol, using a cotton swab or another appropriate method. The diaper should be positioned below the cord to allow it to air dry and to prevent urine from getting on the cord. The nurse should instruct the parents to sponge bathe the infant until the cord falls off. Soap and water shouldn't be used as a part of cord care. Parents should also be instructed to never pull on the cord, but to allow it to fall off naturally. Antibiotic ointments are contraindicated unless there are signs of infection.

Category: Safe and Effective Care Environment: Safety and Infection Control
Subcategory: Pediatrics

44. a. An infant who is admitted with severe diarrhea should be placed in isolation/private room until the cause of diarrhea has been determined. Many causes of diarrhea are very infectious. Choice **b** is incorrect. The infant should be placed in a private room, whether close to the nurse's station or not. Choice **c** is incorrect. The infant should be placed in a private room, not in a room with another infant, since the cause of the diarrhea may be infectious and not shared by the other baby with diarrhea. Choice **d** is incorrect. The infant should be placed in a private room, not in a room with another infant, since the cause of the diarrhea may be infectious.

Category: Safe and Effective Care Environment: Safety and Infection Control
Subcategory: Pediatrics

45. c. The infant should be placed in the back seat in a rear-facing infant car seat. Choice **a** is incorrect. While the infant should use a rear-facing car seat, it should be placed in the back seat. Choice **b** is incorrect. The infant should not be placed in either a forward-facing car seat or the front seat. Choice **d** is incorrect. While the infant should be placed in the back seat, it should be in a rear-facing infant car seat.

Category: Safe and Effective Care Environment: Safety and Infection Control
Subcategory: Maternal Infant: Neonate

46. b. Symptoms of post-traumatic stress disorder include difficulty concentrating and maintaining close relationships. Choice **a** is incorrect. While symptoms of post-traumatic stress disorder include difficulty concentrating, they do not include continuous discussion of the event, which in fact PTSD clients avoid. Choice **c** is incorrect. While symptoms of post-traumatic stress disorder include difficulty maintaining close relationships, repetitive behaviors are a symptom of obsessive-compulsive disorders. Choice **d** is incorrect. The client with post-traumatic stress disorder will tend to avoid discussion of the traumatic event. Repetitive behaviors are a symptom of obsessive-compulsive disorders.

Category: Psychosocial Integrity
Subcategory: Mental Health: Post Traumatic Stress

47. d. A detailed neurovascular assessment is the priority. CMS (circulation/color, movement, and sensation) of the extremity must be checked. Circulation checks include adequate capillary refill through the observation of warm, pink toes. Motion checks requiring the client to move the toe is another priority, as are sensation checks requiring the client to identify touch. Choice **a** is incorrect. Pain upon movement is an expected finding. Choice **b** is incorrect. Inspection of the cast for drainage is important, but not the priority. Choice **c** is incorrect. An assessment of the client's VS is important, but not the priority.
Category: Physiological Integrity: Reduction of Risk
Subcategory: Musculoskeletal Disorders

48. c. Pregnant clients should consume no more than 300 mg of caffeine per day. Choice **a** is incorrect. Caffeine intake of 100 mg per day is not harmful to the client or fetus; current guidelines recommend that pregnant women can consume up to 300 mg of caffeine per day. Choice **b** is incorrect. Caffeine intake of 200 mg per day is not harmful to the client or fetus; current guidelines recommend that pregnant women can consume up to 300 mg of caffeine per day. Choice **d** is incorrect. Consuming more than 300 mg of caffeine per day may increase the health risks for the fetus; therefore, current guidelines recommend that pregnant women consume no more than 300 mg of caffeine per day.
Category: Health Promotion and Maintenance
Subcategory: Maternal Infant: Antepartum

49. The correct answer is a *nomogram*, represented here. The method for determining body surface area is a three-column chart called a nomogram. The nurse marks the child's height in the first column and weight in the third column, then draws a line between the two marks. The point at which the line intersects the vertical scale in the second column indicates the estimated body surface area of the child in square meters.

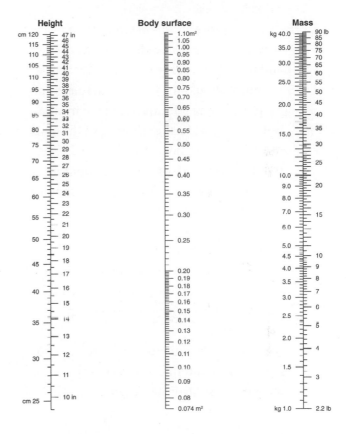

Category: Safe and Effective Care Environment: Safety and Infection Control
Subcategory: Pediatrics

50. d. The calculation is as follows:
$$\frac{1}{1} = \frac{0.5}{x}$$
$$1x = 0.5$$
$$x = 0.5 \text{ mL}$$
Category: Physiological Integrity: Pharmacology
Subcategory: Respiratory Disorders

51. a. The nurse is aware the AIDS virus is caused by HIV. The HIV virus is spread through bodily secretions. The razor should not be shared because it could come in contact with the client's blood and infect other family members with the virus. Choices **b**, **c**, and **d** pose no threat to the family.

Category: Safe and Effective Care Environment: Safety and Infection Control

Subcategory: Medical Surgical: Miscellaneous

52. The correct answer is *apical pulse*.

Because digoxin can reduce the heart rate and heart failure may cause a pulse deficit, the nurse should measure the toddler's apical pulse before administering the medication to prevent further slowing of the heart rate. The medication should be held if the toddler's heart rate is below 120 bpm.

Category: Safe and Effective Care Environment: Safety and Infection Control

Subcategory: Pediatrics

53. The correct answer is a *surgical mask*.

The client requires droplet precautions to prevent spreading the pneumonia to others during the transport to the radiology department.

Category: Safe and Effective Care Environment: Safety and Infection Control

Subcategory: Medical Surgical: Miscellaneous

54. The correct answer is *2, 1, 3, 4, 5*.

In a contact isolation situation, the procedure for the removal of protective gear/wear to prevent cross-contamination is as follows: First, remove one glove by grasping the cuff and pulling the glove inside out over the hand. Discard the glove. With the ungloved hand, tuck a finger inside the cuff of the remaining glove and pull it off, inside out. Next, the eyewear/face shield or goggles should be removed. The gown is removed next. The nurse should untie the waist and neck strings of the gown. Allow the gown to fall from the shoulders. Remove hands from the sleeves without touching the outside of the gown. Hold the gown inside at shoulder seams and fold inside out. Discard in the laundry bag if fabric or in the trash can if the gown is disposable. Remove the mask next without touching the outer surface. Last, the nurse should perform hand hygiene for no less than 15 seconds.

Category: Safe and Effective Care Environment: Safety and Infection Control

Subcategory: Medical Surgical: Miscellaneous

55. a. The infant will feel most comfortable and secure if he or she is being held by the mother during the exam. Choice **b** is incorrect. Most infants are comforted by pacifier use. Therefore, the infant should be allowed to utilize the pacifier during the exam. Choice **c** is incorrect. Infants begin to fear strangers around 9 months. Because of this and because infants are comforted by their mothers, the mother should continue to hold the infant, not give the infant to the nurse. Choice **d** is incorrect. The nurse should not have the mother place the infant on the exam table. Most of the exam can be done with the mother holding the infant to promote the infant's sense of security and comfort.
Category: Physiological Integrity: Basic Care and Comfort
Subcategory: Pediatrics: Assessment

56. d. The chamber that is most likely the source of the fragmented clot responsible for the stroke is the left ventricle (4). Clients diagnosed with atrial fibrillation are at an increased risk for clot formation in the left ventricle. If a piece of the clot dislodges/breaks loose and travels to the client's brain, the client will suffer an embolic stroke. Choice **a** is incorrect. This is the right ventricle; the left ventrical is the site associated with atrial fibrillation. Choice **b** is incorrect. This is the right atrium; the left ventrical is the site associated with atrial fibrillation. Choice **c** is incorrect. This is the left atrium; the left ventrical is the site associated with atrial fibrillation.
Category: Physiological Integrity: Physiological Adaptation
Subcategory: Cardiovascular Disorders

57. a. Barrier cream application will soothe the infant's skin and protect it from further irritation from stool and urine. Choice **b** is incorrect. The infant's buttocks should be cleansed with each diaper change. Choice **c** is incorrect. Exposing the infant's diaper area to air several minutes each day will promote healing of the diaper rash. Choice **d** is incorrect. Yeast ointment should be applied only if the infant has a yeast infection.
Category: Physiological Integrity: Basic Care and Comfort
Subcategory: Pediatrics: Integumentary

58. b. The nurse should encourage the client to discuss the events surrounding the onset of the delusion as this may lead to a discovery of the delusion's trigger. Choice **a** is incorrect. The nurse should not encourage the client's delusion. Choice **c** is incorrect. The nurse should avoid arguing the reality of the delusion with the client. Choice **d** is incorrect. By telling the client that the Tooth Fairy is not real, the nurse is facilitating an argument with the client about the reality of the delusion, something that should be avoided.
Category: Psychosocial Integrity
Subcategory: Mental Health: Delusional Disorders

59. c. +3 edema shows as a 6 mm pit and takes 10 to 12 seconds to rebound. Choice **a** is incorrect. +1 edema shows as a 2 mm, barely detectable pit and rebounds immediately. Choice **b** is incorrect. +2 edema shows as a 4 mm pit and rebounds in a few seconds. Choice **d** is incorrect. +4 edema shows as an 8 mm-or-greater pit and takes more than 20 seconds to rebound.
Category: Health Promotion and Maintenance
Subcategory: Maternal Infant: Antepartum

60. d. Clients in the denial phase express the belief that this could not be happening to their infant or that everything will be fine with their newborn. Choice **a** is incorrect. Clients in the acceptance stage would express the ability to deal with an infant with Dandy-Walker syndrome, a congenital malformation of the brain. Choice **b** is incorrect. Clients in the anger stage would express feelings of anger about the baby having Dandy-Walker syndrome, a congenital malformation of the brain. Choice **c** is incorrect. Clients in the bargaining stage express the willingness to trade almost anything for the health of the infant with a congenital malformation of the brain.

Category: Psychosocial Integrity

Subcategory: Maternal Infant: Newborn Complications

61. The correct answer is *meconium*.

The neonate's first stool is known as the meconium stool. It is tarry and dark green or black in appearance.

Category: Physiological Integrity: Basic Care and Comfort

Subcategory: Maternal Infant: Neonate Assessment

62. a. It is common for pulmonary complications such as atelectasis to develop 24 to 48 hours postoperatively. Choice **b** is incorrect. A fever due to a bladder infection is likely to occur 48 to 72 hours after surgery. Choice **c** is incorrect. A low-grade fever related to dehydration usually occurs in the first 24 hours following surgery. Choice **d** is incorrect. It takes at least 72 hours or longer for a wound infection to develop and cause a fever.

Category: Physiological Integrity: Reduction of Risk

Subcategory: Miscellaneous

63. d. The mother should use a cool mist humidifier in the bedroom of the child with croup, not a dehumidifier. Choice **a** is incorrect. Placing a child in a steamy bathroom can relieve croup symptoms. Choice **b** is incorrect. Increasing the child's fluid intake decreases the child's risk for dehydration from croup. Choice **c** is incorrect. Taking the child out in the cool air can relieve croup symptoms.

Category: Physiological Integrity: Basic Care and Comfort

Subcategory: Pediatrics: Respiratory

64. The correct answer is *3, 4, 1, 2*.

The nurse will respond to this situation utilizing the RACE mnemonic; Rescue, Alarm, Confine, Extinguish.

Category: Safe and Effective Care Environment: Safety and Infection Control

Subcategory: Medical Surgical: Miscellaneous

65. d. The nurse needs to recognize that thrombocytopenia alters coagulation; it poses a high risk/potential of bleeding. To help prevent capillary bleeding, the nurse should use the smallest needle possible when administering any type of injection. Choice **a** is incorrect. The nurse should record accurate intake and output to monitor hydration; however, this nursing action/intervention does not protect the client from a complication associated with thrombocytopenia. Choice **b** is incorrect. The nurse should provide comfort measures and maintain the client on bed rest as ordered; activities such as using a wheelchair can cause injury and bleeding. Choice **c** is incorrect. The nurse doesn't need to limit visits by family members or friends because they do not pose any danger to the client.

Category: Safe and Effective Care Environment: Safety and Infection Control

Subcategory: Medical Surgical: Oncology Disorders

66. a. The nurse should first place the client in the high-Fowler's position, with the head of the bed raised. After placing the client in the high-Fowler's position and moving the client to the side of the bed, the nurse helps the client sit on the edge of the bed and dangle his or her legs to prevent a sudden drop in BP upon standing/moving (inducing orthostatic hypotension). The nurse should then face the client and place the chair next to and facing the head of the bed. Choice **b** is incorrect. This is incorrect technique. The nurse would not be able to assist the client from behind. Choice **c** is incorrect. This is incorrect technique. The nurse should face the chair toward the head, not the foot, of the bed, since the raised head of the bed can provide some support as the client moves to the wheelchair. Choice **d** is incorrect. This is incorrect technique. The head of the bed should be raised to allow the patient extra support during the transfer to the wheelchair.
Category: Safe and Effective Care Environment: Safety and Infection Control
Subcategory: Medical Surgical: Miscellaneous

67. b. The digoxin should be held 24 to 72 hours prior to the elective cardioversion. A client on digoxin is more prone to rhythm problems at the time of the shock, especially if the level in the blood is high. Holding the digoxin tends to reduce the incidence of such problems. Diuretics are also held. Choice **a** is incorrect. Coumadin, an anticoagulant, does not need to be held, as cardioversion does not increase the risk for bleeding. Choice **c** is incorrect. Heparin, an anticoagulant, does not need to be held, as cardioversion does not increase the risk for bleeding. Choice **d** is incorrect. Valium is generally used for a sedative effect during an elective cardioversion and should not be held; the dosage and route should be adjusted if the physician orders an adjustment.
Category: Physiological Integrity: Pharmacology
Subcategory: Cardiovascular Disorders

68. d. This option/practice prevents surgical asepsis. Choice **a** is incorrect. This option/practice aids in ensuring surgical asepsis. Consider $1\frac{1}{2}$ inches around the edge of a sterile field to be contaminated. Do NOT place anything sterile in that area. Choice **b** is incorrect. This option/practice aids in ensuring surgical asepsis. The sterile field ends at the level of the tabletop or at the waist of the sterile person's gown. Choice **c** is incorrect. This option/practice aids in ensuring surgical asepsis. This assures the flap will not come in contact with the nurse.
Category: Safe and Effective Care Environment: Safety and Infection Control
Subcategory: Medical Surgical: Miscellaneous

69. b. The terminal ileum of the small intestines is the part of the intestines brought to the abdominal surface in ileostomies. Choice **a** is incorrect. Site A is the ascending colon and is the part of the intestines brought to the abdominal surface in ascending colostomies. Choice **c** is incorrect. This is the transverse colon, the part of the intestines brought to the abdominal surface in transverse colostomies. Choice **d** is incorrect. This is the descending colon, the part of the intestines brought to the abdominal surface in descending colostomies.
Category: Physiological Integrity: Physiological Adaptation
Subcategory: Pediatrics: Gastrointestinal

70. a. The client is having difficulty swallowing. The client is at the greatest risk for developing aspiration pneumonia. Choice **b** is incorrect. The client with this diagnosis could develop bladder distension, but in this scenario the client is at the greatest risk for developing aspiration pneumonia. Choice **c** is incorrect. Decubitus ulcers may occur, but in this scenario the client is at the greatest risk for developing aspiration pneumonia. Choice **d** is incorrect. Hypertensive crisis is not likely to occur in a client with this diagnosis.
Category: Physiological Integrity: Reduction of Risk
Subcategory: Musculoskeletal Disorders

71. c. To perform the Weber's test, the tuning fork should be struck and then placed on the midline of the client's head, as shown here. The Weber's test aids in determining whether sound is heard equally in both ears. If the client hears the sound louder in one ear, he or she probably has unequal hearing loss that requires further evaluation and intervention.

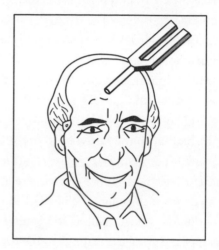

Category: Health Promotion and Maintenance
Subcategory: Medical Surgical: Sensory Disorders

72. c. The HITS screening tool consists of four questions that screen for domestic violence. Each question is scored on a scale of 1 to 5. A total score of 10 or greater is considered to be positive. Choice **a** is incorrect. The SKIN scale determines risk for skin breakdown/pressure ulcers. Choice **b** is incorrect. A BSE is a screening tool for breast cancer. Choice **d** is incorrect. The PSA test is a screening tool for prostate cancer.
Category: Psychosocial Integrity
Subcategory: Mental Health: Abuse

73. a. It is recommended that clients consume fluids one half hour before and/or after meals versus water with meals to decrease symptoms of morning sickness. Choice **b** is incorrect. Eating dry crackers or cereal before getting out of bed in the morning can help to decrease the symptoms of morning sickness. Choice **c** is incorrect. Eating small, frequent meals throughout the day can decrease the symptoms of morning sickness. Choice **d** is incorrect. Eating foods that are bland can help to decrease the symptoms of morning sickness.

Category: Physiological Integrity: Basic Care and Comfort

Subcategory: Maternal Infant: Antepartum

74. b. The neonate should take both the nipple and as much of the lower portion of the areola as possible into its mouth. Choice **a** is incorrect. If the neonate's lips are located on the breast tissue, the neonate would have too much of the breast in its mouth to feed effectively. Choice **c** is incorrect. The neonate should take the entire nipple and as much of the lower portion of the areola as possible into its mouth. Choice **d** is incorrect. The neonate's lips should rest on the areola as well as the nipple.

Category: Physiological Integrity: Basic Care and Comfort

Subcategory: Maternal Infant: Breastfeeding

75. c. Mongolian spots are large blue or blue-gray birthmarks that appear near the buttocks at birth or shortly after. Choice **a** is incorrect. Large blue or blue-gray marks that appear near the buttocks at birth or shortly after are not the result of abuse but are birthmarks known as Mongolian spots. Choice **b** is incorrect. Milia present as tiny white bumps on the cheeks, nose, and chin of the newborn. Choice **d** is incorrect. Montgomery tubercles are tiny white spots that occur in the areola.

Category: Physiological Integrity: Physiological Adaptation

Subcategory: Maternal Infant: Neonate

76. a. Easing the client to a sitting position on the floor is the priority action. This will help prevent the client from falling and will keep the client safe. Choice **b** is incorrect. Having the client place her head between her legs will not keep her from falling. Choice **c** is incorrect. This is unsafe. Encouraging the client to walk faster will likely intensify the dizziness and the client's fainting sensation. Choice **d** is incorrect. The nurse should never leave a client who is complaining of dizziness and feeling faint.

Category: Physiological Integrity: Reduction of Risk

Subcategory: Neurological Disorders

77. d. The pedal pulse is located on the top of the foot. Choice **a** is incorrect. The pedal pulse is located on the top of the foot, not on the side of the ankle. Choice **b** is incorrect. The pedal pulse is located on the top of the foot, not on the side of the heel. Choice **c** is incorrect. The pedal pulse is located on the top of the foot, not on the side of the foot.

Category: Health Promotion and Maintenance

Subcategory: Medical Surgical: Miscellaneous

78. c. The client should be instructed to refrain from eating cantaloupe, fish, and turnips, as well as red meat, for 48 to 72 hours before the test and throughout the collection process. The client should be encouraged to maintain a high-fiber diet which will aid in increasing stool volume and decreasing colonic transit time and intraluminal pressure, thus preventing constipation.
Category: Health Promotion and Maintenance
Subcategory: Medical Surgical: Oncology Disorders

79. b. The nurse should instruct the client to splint the incision with a pillow to decrease the discomfort associated with coughing and deep breathing. Choice **a** is incorrect. This is inappropriate; the nurse may try to schedule the coughing and breathing exercises after the client has received pain medication. Choice **c** is incorrect. Coughing and deep breathing exercises should occur every two hours; waiting four hours is not the best option. Choice **d** is incorrect. This is a true statement, but inappropriate.
Category: Physiological Integrity: Reduction of Risk
Subcategory: Respiratory Disorders

80. b. The nurse should measure the abdominal girth at the umbilicus in order to obtain the most accurate measurement. Using any other location would not produce an accurate measurement. Choices **a** and **d** are incorrect. The nurse should measure the abdominal girth at the umbilicus in order to obtain the most accurate measurement. These locations are above the umbilicus. Choice **c** is incorrect. This location is below the umbilicus.
Category: Health Promotion and Maintenance
Subcategory: Medical Surgical: Gastrointestinal Disorders

81. c. The nurse should administer the injection in the vastuslateralis muscle. Choice **a** is incorrect. The deltoid muscle should not be used to administer IM injections until a child is 3 years old. Choice **b** is incorrect. The dorsogluteal muscle is not well developed and is not the best choice for administering an IM injection in the newborn. Choice **d** is incorrect. The rectus femoris muscle is not well developed in the newborn and therefore is not the best choice for administering an IM injection.
Category: Physiological Integrity: Pharmacology
Subcategory: Maternal Infant: Neonate

82. b. Aspirin at low dosages (81 mg) can reduce the potential for developing a blood clot, which could occlude the narrowed opening in a diseased coronary artery. This antiplatelet effect is used to prevent blood clot formation inside arteries, particularly in individuals who have atherosclerosis or are otherwise prone to develop blood clots in their arteries. Choice **a** is incorrect. Aspirin will relieve headaches and muscle pain. Choice **c** is incorrect. Aspirin will not lower blood pressure. Choice **d** is incorrect. Aspirin does not dilate the coronary arteries.
Category: Physiological Integrity: Pharmacology
Subcategory: Cardiovascular Disorders

83. b. The nurse would expect a client with anticipatory anxiety to fear what will happen next. Choice **a** is incorrect. Fear that is constantly present is associated with free-floating anxiety. Choice **c** is incorrect. Mistrust and suspicion of others is associated with paranoid personality disorder. Choice **d** is incorrect. A sense of impending doom is associated with panic disorder.
Category: Psychosocial Integrity
Subcategory: Mental Health: Anxiety

84. The answer is *5.59 centimeters.*
To convert from inches to centimeters, multiply the length in inches by 2.54. In this example, 2.2 is multiplied by 2.54 to get 5.59 centimeters.
Category: Physiological Integrity: Basic Care and Comfort
Subcategory: Maternal Infant: Integumentary

85. b. The nurse should make certain that the client has a PSA test completed prior to a rectal examination. A client may have falsely high levels of PSA for up to 12 days after a rectal examination or instrumentation around the prostate gland, such as occurs during a cystoscopy. Choices **a**, **c**, and **d** are tests not influenced by a rectal examination.
Category: Health Promotion and Maintenance
Subcategory: Medical Surgical: Oncology Disorders

86. b. Oliguria and tinnitus are symptoms of acetylsalicylic acid (aspirin) overdose. Choice **a** is incorrect. Both jaundice and abdominal pain are symptoms of acetaminophen (Tylenol) overdose. Choice **c** is incorrect. While tinnitus is a symptom of acetylsalicylic acid (aspirin) overdose, jaundice is a symptom of acetaminophen (Tylenol) overdose. Choice **d** is incorrect. While oliguria is a symptom of acetylsalicylic acid (aspirin) overdose, abdominal pain is a symptom of acetaminophen (Tylenol) overdose.
Category: Physiological Integrity: Physiological Adaptation
Subcategory: Pediatrics: Poisoning

87. d. Pernicious anemia is a lack of vitamin B12 often caused by a lack of intrinsic factor in the GI tract. Intrinsic factor is necessary for the absorption of B12. A lack of B12 can cause peripheral neuropathy. Other signs and symptoms of pernicious anemia include: diarrhea or constipation; fatigue; lack of energy, or lightheadedness when standing up or with exertion; loss of appetite; pale skin; problems concentrating; shortness of breath, mostly during exercise; swollen, red tongue or bleeding gums; confusion; depression; and loss of balance. Choice **a** is incorrect. An increased appetite is not associated with pernicious anemia. Choice **b** is incorrect. A decreased platelet count is not associated with pernicious anemia. Choice **c** is incorrect. Ecchymosis is not associated with pernicious anemia.
Category: Physiological Integrity: Reduction of Risk
Subcategory: Hematological Disorders

88. a. The classic location of pain from appendicitis occurs in the right lower quadrant of the abdomen. Choice **b** is incorrect. This is the upper right quadrant of the abdomen and may be the site of pain related to gallbladder or liver disease but it is not the classic site of pain from appendicitis. Choice **c** is incorrect. This is the upper left quadrant of the abdomen and may be the site of pain related to diverticulitis but it is not the classic site of pain from appendicitis. Choice **d** is incorrect. This is the lower left quadrant. This may be the site of pain related to inflammatory bowel disease but it is not the classic site of pain from appendicitis.
Category: Physiological Integrity: Physiological Adaptation
Subcategory: Pediatrics: Gastrointestinal

89. a. Screening for lead poisoning consists of an assessment of blood levels of lead and is generally completed between the ages of 1 and 2 (earlier in high-risk areas). Choice **b** is incorrect. While children with lead poisoning can experience bone pain, bone X-rays cannot detect the presence of lead in the blood. Choice **c** is incorrect. Chelation therapy is a treatment for lead poisoning. Choice **d** is incorrect. While kidney function is impacted by lead poisoning, the screening required is for blood levels of lead.
Category: Physiological Integrity: Reduction of Risk Potential
Subcategory: Pediatrics: Poisoning

90. c. The nurse should discourage the client from restricting fluids because this can lead to a fluid imbalance. Restricting fluids can also lead to more concentrated urine and stone formation. Choices **a** and **b** are incorrect. It is unsafe to encourage the client to restrict fluids. Choice **d** is incorrect. Inadequate fluid intake does not contribute to constipation.
Category: Health Promotion and Maintenance
Subcategory: Medical Surgical: Neurological Disorders

91. c. Having the client insert a tampon or sterile gauze square into the stoma while changing the appliance will temporarily absorb the dripping urine and aid in keeping the client's skin dry. Choice **a** is incorrect. Leaning over the toilet to permit urine to drip in the toilet puts the client in an awkward position during the appliance change. Choices **b** and **d** are incorrect. Both hands are needed to complete the appliance change.
Category: Health Promotion and Maintenance
Subcategory: Medical Surgical: Gastrointestinal Disorders

92. c. Hepatitis A is caused by infection with the hepatitis A virus. The hepatitis virus is usually spread when a person ingests tiny amounts of contaminated fecal matter. Hepatitis A virus can be transmitted several ways, such as: when someone with the virus handles the food you eat without first carefully washing his or her hands after using the toilet; drinking contaminated water; and eating raw shellfish from water polluted with sewage. Choice **a** is incorrect. Hepatitis C is usually caused by contact with infected blood, including receiving blood transfusions. Choice **b** is incorrect. Hepatitis C is usually caused by contact with infected blood, including receiving blood transfusions. Choice **d** is incorrect. Hepatitis B is caused by blood and sexual contact with an infected person.
Category: Health Promotion and Maintenance
Subcategory: Medical Surgical: Gastrointestinal Disorders

93. d. The client experiencing a manic episode experiences decreased appetite and a tendency to forget to eat, and therefore experiences weight loss. Choice **a** is incorrect. The client experiencing a manic episode experiences a sense of inflated, not decreased, self-esteem. Choice **b** is incorrect. The client experiencing a manic episode experiences decreased, not increased, sleep. Choice **c** is incorrect. The client experiencing a manic episode has a decreased, not increased, appetite.
Category: Psychosocial Integrity
Subcategory: Mental Health: Bipolar Disorder

94. c. Panic attacks typically include a few or many of the following symptoms: sense of impending doom or danger, fear of loss of control or death, tachycardia, sweating, trembling, shortness of breath, hyperventilation, chills, hot flashes, abdominal cramping, nausea, diarrhea (GI distress), chest pains, headache, dizziness, faintness, tightness in the throat, and rapid speech.
Category: Psychosocial Integrity
Subcategory: Mental Health

95. b. Betamethasone (Celestone) should be administered via the intramuscular route. Choice **a** is incorrect. Betamethasone (Celestone) should be administered via the intramuscular route, not orally. Choice **c** is incorrect. Betamethasone (Celestone) should be administered via the intramuscular route, not intravenously. Choice **d** is incorrect. Betamethasone (Celestone) should be administered via the intramuscular route, not sublingually.
Category: Physiological Integrity: Pharmacology
Subcategory: Maternal Infant: Medication Administration

96. The answer is *front* to *back*.
Wiping from front to back decreases the risk for microorganisms to enter into the urinary tract.
Category: Physiological Integrity: Reduction of Risk Potential
Subcategory: Pediatrics: Genitourinary

97. c. Obesity is a risk factor for gestational diabetes. Choice **a** is incorrect. While alcohol consumption is contraindicated during pregnancy, it is not a risk factor for gestational diabetes. Choice **b** is incorrect. Maternal age greater, not less, than 35 is a risk factor for gestational diabetes. Choice **d** is incorrect. Gestational diabetes can lead to preterm labor but preterm labor is not a risk factor for gestational diabetes.

Category: Physiological Integrity: Reduction of Risk Potential

Subcategory: Maternal Infant: Antepartum

98. c. The nurse correctly suspects infection when the amniotic fluid is yellow in color. Choice **a** is incorrect. If the client were experiencing placental abruption, the amniotic fluid would be port-wine in color. Choice **b** is incorrect. If the fetus were experiencing fetal distress, the amniotic fluid would be green or black in color from meconium stool. Choice **d** is incorrect. Normal amniotic fluid is clear or clear with white flecks.

Category: Physiological Integrity: Reduction of Risk Potential

Subcategory: Maternal Infant: Intrapartum

99. c. The use of cocaine can induce cardiac dysrhythmias, and toxicity may occur anytime and with any dose. Other associated symptoms include chest pains and death. Choice **a** is incorrect. The client would experience an increased heart rate, not bradycardia, a decreased or slow heart rate. Choice **b** is incorrect. The client's blood glucose levels may decrease. Choice **d** is incorrect. The client's respirations would be increased.

Category: Psychosocial Integrity

Subcategory: Mental Health

100. c. MS is thought to be an autoimmune disease/disorder. Choice **a** is incorrect. The West Nile virus enecephalitis, not MS, is associated with bites from mosquitoes that are infected. Choice **b** is incorrect. Shingles, not MS, occurs in people who have had chickenpox in the past. Choice **d** is incorrect. Commonly, acute glomerulonephritis and rheumatic fever, not MS, follow a streptococcal infection.

Category: Physiological Integrity: Physiological Adaptation

Subcategory: Musculoskeletal Disorders

101. b. Platelets are administered when client bleeding is associated with deficient platelet count or function, not hemophilia A. Choice **a** is incorrect. Froze factor VIII (cryoprecipitate) is administered to patients with hemophilia A. Choice **c** is incorrect. Joints impacted by hemophilia A should be immobilized and elevated, with ice applied to the site. Choice **d** is incorrect. It is appropriate to implement bleeding precautions for clients with hemophilia A.

Category: Physiological Integrity: Reduction of Risk Potential

Subcategory: Pediatrics: Hematological

102. d. The most common sign of marijuana usage is inflammation of the eyes (2) and a rapid pulse (6). There is no evidence that marijuana use increases a client's sexual drive (1). Pinpoint pupils (3) are a sign of heroin usage. Restlessness (4) is associated with abrupt alcohol withdrawal. Shivering (5) is seen with opiate withdrawal. Other signs of marijuana use are: drowsiness, euphoria, hunger, and lightheadedness.

Category: Psychosocial Integrity

Subcategory: Mental Health

103. d. The nurse should check the PTT. The PTT is utilized to monitor a client's response to heparin therapy. The therapeutic range is 1.5 to 2.0 times the control time. Choice **a** is incorrect. The CBC reports the number of blood cells, not clotting factors. Choice **b** is incorrect. Hemoglobin relates to the blood's oxygen carrying capacity and is unaffected by heparin therapy. Choice **c** is incorrect. PT is used to monitor a client's response to oral anticoagulants.

Category: Physiological Integrity: Pharmacology

Subcategory: Cardiovascular Disorders

104. d. Jelly does not contain phenylalanine and can be consumed by children with PKU. Choice **a** is incorrect. Aspartame contains nearly 50% phenylalanine and should be avoided by children with PKU. Choice **b** is incorrect. Fish is high in protein and therefore high in phenylalanine and should be avoided by children with PKU. Choice **c** is incorrect. Ice cream and dairy products contain high levels of phenylalanine and should be avoided by children with PKU.

Category: Physiological Integrity: Reduction of Risk Potential

Subcategory: Pediatrics: Endocrine

105. a. Clients with esophageal atresia are at high risk for aspiration. Choice **b** is incorrect. Clients with esophageal atresia are at high risk for aspiration and therefore should be kept NPO. Choice **c** is incorrect. Clients with esophageal atresia are at high risk for aspiration and therefore should have the heads of their beds elevated. Choice **d** is incorrect. Tracheal suction is performed when clients cannot cough and clear their own secretions from their air passages. Clients with esophageal atresia are able to cough but have copious amounts of mouth secretions that may require suctioning of the mouth.

Category: Physiological Integrity: Reduction of Risk Potential

Subcategory: Pediatrics: Gastrointestinal

106. b. The nurse should encourage the client to express his feelings; this is very therapeutic. Clients with PTSD who are able to remember the precipitating traumatic event use a lot of energy to control their feelings and/or suppress the memory of it; thus, permitting the client to express his feelings would be the most beneficial. Choice **a** is incorrect. Administering antianxiety medications may be necessary, but encouraging the client to express his feelings is most therapeutic. Choice **c** is incorrect. Monitoring the client's physical symptoms may be necessary, but encouraging the client to express his feelings is most therapeutic. Choice **d** is incorrect. Observing the client's interactions with family and friends might be useful, but encouraging the client to express his feelings is most therapeutic.

Category: Psychosocial Integrity

Subcategory: Mental Health

107. c. When a client displays anxiety and/or is worried or fearful, the nurse should encourage the client to express his or her feelings and listen attentively. Choice **a** is incorrect. This is an inappropriate intervention. The nurse should engage the client in communication. Avoiding the subject displays uncaring behavior. Choice **b** is incorrect. This is inappropriate and will not aid in relieving the client's anxiety. Choice **d** is incorrect. This is an inappropriate intervention. The client's ability to learn is impaired during times of crisis.

Category: Psychosocial Integrity
Subcategory: Medical Surgical: Cardiovascular Disorders

108. a. Signs of alcohol withdrawal occur within the first 48 hours of admission and include headaches, anxiety, shaky feeling, hand tremors, seizures, and elevated heart rate. Choice **b** is incorrect. Blood pressure is an assessment for hypertension and hypotension. The client is not experiencing symptoms of hypotension or hypertension such as lightheadedness, headaches, or dizziness. Choice **c** is incorrect. Hemoglobin A1c is used to assess how well a client's diabetes is being controlled over time. Choice **d** is incorrect. While a medication assessment is important, given the fact that the client is experiencing symptoms of withdrawal, it is more important to find out the client's alcohol consumption patterns.

Category: Psychosocial Integrity
Subcategory: Mental Health: Chemical Dependency

109. b. Involuntary writhing motions are associated with athetosis. Choice **a** is incorrect. Diminished reflexes are associated with hypotonia. Choice **c** is incorrect. Rigidity is associated with hypertonia. Choice **d** is incorrect. Uncoordinated muscle movement is associated with ataxia.

Category: Physiological Integrity: Physiological Adaptation
Subcategory: Pediatrics: Neurologic

110. c. Loss of personal memories is associated with dissociative amnesia disorder. Choice **a** is incorrect. Alternating periods of euphoria and depression is associated with bipolar disorder. Choice **b** is incorrect. Gradual loss of mental abilities is associated with Alzheimer's disease. Choice **d** is incorrect. Loss of personal reality is associated with depersonalization disorder.

Category: Psychosocial Integrity
Subcategory: Mental Health: Dissociative Disorder

111. d. Clients who are in unfamiliar circumstances/environments require information about hospital equipment, procedures, and routines. Providing this information will best aid in relieving the client's anxiety. Choice **a** is incorrect. This intervention is not appropriate in this situation. Choices **b** and **c** are incorrect. These will not relieve the client's anxiety and may actually intensify it.

Category: Psychosocial Integrity
Subcategory: Medical Surgical: Cardiovascular Disorders

112. b. Pounds are converted to kilograms by dividing by 2.2. 43 divided by 2.2 equals 19.5.

Category: Physiological Integrity: Pharmacology
Subcategory: Pediatrics: Medication Administration

113. b. Nonverbal cues may have different meanings in different cultures. The nurse should always respect the client's cultural beliefs and ask whether he or she has cultural requirements. These may include food choices or restrictions, body coverings, or time for prayer. The nurse should attempt to understand the client's culture; it is not the client's responsibility to understand the nurse's culture. The nurse should never impose her own beliefs on her clients. Culture influences a client's experience with pain.
Category: Psychosocial Integrity
Subcategory: Medical Surgical: Miscellaneous

114. d. The best therapeutic approach is for the nurse to reflect on the client's comment, focusing on his or her specific words. Choice **a** is incorrect. This statement offers false reassurance and ignores the client's needs. Choice **b** is incorrect. Telling the client he or she is doing well is a nontherapeutic response. This statement offers false reassurance and ignores the client's needs. Choice **c** is incorrect. Telling the client that special equipment is available is a nontherapeutic response. This statement offers false reassurance and ignores the client's needs.
Category: Psychosocial Integrity
Subcategory: Medical Surgical: Miscellaneous

115. c. The calculation is as follows:
$$\frac{\text{desired dose}}{\text{dosage available}} \times \text{total quantity} = \text{dose}$$
$$\frac{10}{20} \times 1 \text{ tablet} = 0.5 \text{ tablet}$$
Category: Physiological Integrity: Pharmacology
Subcategory: Oncology Disorders

116. a. To administer eardrops, the nurse should gently pull the pinna down and back. Choice **b** is incorrect. While the nurse should pull the pinna gently down, it should not be pulled out. Choice **c** is incorrect. While the nurse should pull the pinna gently backward, the pinna should be down versus up. Choice **d** is incorrect. The nurse should gently pull the pinna up and out for older children and adults.
Category: Physiological Integrity: Pharmacology
Subcategory: Pediatrics: Medication Administration

117. c. Insulin levels are not decreased/reduced by hemodialysis. Choice **a** is incorrect. The hemodialysis treatment will not destroy the injected insulin. Choice **b** is incorrect. The hemodialysis treatment does not stimulate insulin production. Choice **d** is incorrect. Insulin will not enhance the effects of the hemodialysis treatment.
Category: Physiological Integrity: Physiological Adaptation
Subcategory: Endocrine Disorders

118. d. For an accurate comparison, the client should be weighed at the same time daily, with similar clothing, on the same scale. Choice **a** is incorrect. The client's normal/predisease weight has no bearing on the current situation and condition except as a point of reference. Choice **b** is incorrect. Not all clients need to be weighed on a bedside scale. Choice **c** is incorrect. There is nothing in this scenario that states whether the client wore footwear during previous weight assessments.
Category: Physiological Integrity: Basic Care and Comfort
Subcategory: Medical Surgical: Renal Disorders

119. d. A lithium level of 1.9 mEq/L is within the toxic range. Symptoms of lithium toxicity include tremors. Choice **a** is incorrect. Agitation is an adverse reaction to medications such as monoamine oxidase (MAO) inhibitors but is not a sign of lithium toxicity. Choice **b** is incorrect. Drooling is a sign of tardive dyskinesia, an adverse reaction to antipsychotic medications. Choice **c** is incorrect. Headaches can be an adverse reaction to benzodiazepines but are not a symptom of toxicity.

Category: Physiological Integrity: Pharmacology

Subcategory: Mental Health: Medication Administration

120. d. Because the client is 30 years old, a bedside commode is most appropriate because the client will probably need no or minimal assistance getting out of the bed. Choice **a** is incorrect. Answering a client call bell promptly is always important, but not critical in this scenario because the client can get up without assistance. Choice **b** is incorrect. Assisting the client to the bathroom often may not be helpful or appropriate. It is most appropriate for a client this age to have a bedside commode, as the client is likely to not need help getting out of bed. Choice **c** is incorrect. Using a disposable brief is emotionally difficult and done only as a last resort.

Category: Physiological Integrity: Basic Care and Comfort

Subcategory: Medical Surgical: Gastrointestinal Disorders

121. a. A bulging fontanel can be indicative of increased intercranial pressure. Choice **b** is incorrect. Cephalohematoma is a benign swelling of the tissues in the newborn's head that is self-resolving. Choice **c** is incorrect. Molding of the infant's head occurs to facilitate movement through the birth canal. It is temporary and self-resolving. Choice **d** is incorrect. The posterior fontanel of the newborn should be open.

Category: Physiolgical Integrity: Reduction of Risk Potential

Subcategory: Maternal Infant: Neonate

122. c. The irrigations will best be completed with the client sitting on the toilet. This position and environment will aid in simulating normal bowel elimination. The stool and irrigation fluid can also be easily flushed down the toilet. Choice **a** is incorrect. This is an unsafe position. Choice **b** is incorrect. This position will not facilitate effective irrigations. Choice **d** is incorrect. This position may be effective, but disposing of the stool and irrigation fluid in the sink may create a problem.

Category: Physiological Integrity: Basic Care and Comfort

Subcategory: Medical Surgical: Gastrointestinal Disorders

123. b. The calculation is as follows:

$$\frac{\text{desired dose}}{\text{dosage available}} \times \text{total quantity} = \text{dose}$$

$$\frac{50}{100} \times 1 \text{ mL} = 0.5 \text{ mL}$$

Category: Physiological Integrity: Pharmacology

Subcategory: Miscellaneous

124. d. The calculation is:

$$x \text{ teaspoons} = \frac{500 \text{ mg}}{1} \times \frac{1 \text{ tsp}}{125 \text{ mg}} = 4 \text{ teaspoons}$$

Choice **a** is incorrect. If the nurse administered 0.25 teaspoons, the child would receive less than the dose ordered. Choice **b** is incorrect. If the nurse administered 2 teaspoons, the child would receive less than the dose ordered. Choice **c** is incorrect. If the nurse administered 3 teaspoons, the child would receive less than the dose ordered.

Category: Physiological Integrity: Pharmacological

Subcategory: Pediatrics: Medication Administration

125. d. This technique helps to remove secretions in all directions within the airway. Choice **a** is incorrect. This is an unacceptable technique for suctioning; the catheter should not be pinched anytime during the procedure. Choice **b** is incorrect. This technique may cause the nurse to exceed the recommended time for suctioning (10 to 15 seconds). Choice **c** is incorrect. This is an unacceptable technique for suctioning; the catheter should not be thrust up or down as this would cause trauma.

Category: Physiological Integrity: Basic Care and Comfort

Subcategory: Medical Surgical: Respiratory Disorders

126. c. A client diagnosed with MS tires easily and requires frequent rest periods. Thus, it is necessary to schedule rest periods between activities to manage symptoms. Choice **a** is incorrect. The client is entitled to have all basic care needs met; if the client is unable to complete all ADLs independently, the nursing staff is responsible. Choice **b** is incorrect. Rushing through tasks/activities will probably tire the client. Choice **d** is incorrect. Completing activities that the client can do is demeaning.

Category: Physiological Integrity: Basic Care and Comfort

Subcategory: Medical Surgical: Neurological Disorders

127. c. The nurse should administer the medication just prior to the child's inhaling to be sure that the maximum amount of medication reaches the child's lungs. Choice **a** is incorrect. If the nurse administers the medication as the child is exhaling, the exhalation will prevent the medication from entering into the lungs. Choice **b** is incorrect. If the nurse administers the medication as the child is inhaling, not all the medication will reach the lungs. Choice **d** is incorrect. If the nurse administers the medication just prior to the child exhaling, the exhalation will prevent the medication from entering the child's lungs.

Category: Physiological Integrity: Pharmacology

Subcategory: Pediatrics: Medication Administration

128. c. Benzodiazepines can cause daytime drowsiness, vertigo, and hypertension, placing an elderly client at risk for falls. Therefore, the plan of care should include implementation of fall precautions. Choice **a** is incorrect. Ativan may cause an adverse reaction of hypotension, not hypertension. Choice **b** is incorrect. Megaloblastic anemia can cause an adverse reaction to barbiturates and sedatives, but not benzodiazepines. Choice **d** is incorrect. The client exhibits no signs/symptoms that place the client at risk for suicide, and benzodiazepines do not increase the risk for suicide. Therefore, suicide precautions are not indicated at this time.

Category: Physiological Integrity: Pharmacology

Subcategory: Mental Health: Medication Administration

129. a. Heart rate and respiratory effort are both assessed when determining the neonate's Apgar score. Choice **b** is incorrect. While respiratory effort is assessed during the determination of the Apgar score, the sucking reflex is not. Choice **c** is incorrect. While the heart rate is assessed during the determination of the Apgar score, urinary output is not. Choice **d** is incorrect. While respiratory effort is assessed during the determination of the Apgar score, urinary output is not.

Category: Physiological Integrity: Reduction of Risk Potential

Subcategory: Maternal Infant: Neonate

130. c. The nurse should encourage the client to consume the majority of fluids in the morning to compensate for the long period without oral fluids while sleeping. Choices **a** and **b** are incorrect. Consuming large amounts of fluid during this time period may cause nocturia and interfere with sleep. Choice **d** is incorrect. Consuming large amounts of fluid after meals may cause gastrointestinal fullness or upset.

Category: Physiological Integrity: Basic Care and Comfort

Subcategory: Medical Surgical: Musculoskeletal Disorders

131. c. When a client is experiencing hypovolemic shock he or she experiences decreased circulating blood volume, and the urinary output decreases. Choice **a** is incorrect. The heart rate would be increased. Choice **b** is incorrect. The respiratory rate would be increased. Choice **d** is incorrect. The systolic and diastolic BP would both decrease.

Category: Physiological Integrity: Physiological Adaptation

Subcategory: Miscellaneous Disorders

132. b. Baclofen's principal clinical indication is for the paraplegic or tetraplegic client with spinal cord lesions, most commonly caused by multiple sclerosis or trauma. Baclofen significantly reduces the number and severity of painful flexor spasms. Choices **a**, **c**, and **d** are incorrect.
Category: Physiological Integrity: Pharmacology
Subcategory: Neurological Disorders

133. c. The suture lines in a 1-year-old child with hydrocephalus would widen due to increased intracranial pressure. Choice **a** is incorrect. A sunken fontanel is indicative of dehydration. In a child with hydrocephalus, the fontanel would be bulging. Choice **b** is incorrect. A child with hydrocephalus would experience lethargy, not increased activity. Choice **d** is incorrect. The blood pressure of a child with hydrocephalus would increase while the pulse decreased due to increased intracranial pressure.
Category: Physiological Integrity: Physiological Adaptation
Subcategory: Pediatrics: Neurological Disorders

134. d. When a client has a cystostomy, a catheter is inserted percutaneously through the suprapubic area into the bladder; this location is where the bladder sits. The nurse would check the suprapubic area for placement. Choice **a** is incorrect. The catheter should be inserted into the bladder; this location is the kidney. Choice **b** is incorrect. The catheter should be inserted into the bladder; this location indicates the ureter. Choice **c** is incorrect. The catheter should be inserted into the bladder; this location indicates the umbilicus.
Category: Physiological Integrity: Basic Care and Comfort
Subcategory: Medical Surgical: Renal Disorders

135. d. The nurse should monitor the client's weight on a daily basis to gauge the response to medical interventions. A significant weight gain or loss indicates changes in fluid distribution (2 lb or more in 24 hours). Weight gain indicates fluid retention and impaired renal excretion. A weight loss indicates a therapeutic response to medical and medication therapy. Choice **a** is incorrect. Appetite is appropriate to assess; however, appetite is not an indicator of heart failure. Appetite is not likely to cause major changes in a client diagnosed with heart failure. Choice **b** is incorrect. Edema of the lower extremities is a sign of right-sided heart failure; also, lower extremities should be assessed more than once daily. Choice **c** is incorrect. Pupil response is appropriate to assess; however, pupil response is not an indicator of heart failure. Pupil response is not likely to cause major changes in a client diagnosed with heart failure.
Category: Physiological Integrity: Basic Care and Comfort
Subcategory: Medical Surgical: Cardiovascular Disorders

136. c. Tolerance occurs when a client needs increasing amounts of a medication/substance to achieve the desired effect. Choice **a** is incorrect. A client is dependent on a medication/substance when he or she has intermittent or continuous cravings for the medication that lead to misuse/abuse. Choice **b** is incorrect. Substance abuse occurs when a client utilizes a medication or substance in amounts or with methods not approved by medical professionals. There is no indication the client is abusing morphine. Choice **d** is incorrect. Withdrawal symptoms occur when a client ceases to utilize a medication/substance.

Category: Physiological Integrity: Pharmacology

Subcategory: Mental Health: Medication Administration

137. d. Prostaglandin E is used on laboring clients to ripen the cervix. Choice **a** is incorrect. Pitocin/oxitocin is the medication utilized to increase uterine contractions in a laboring woman. Choice **b** is incorrect. Magnesium sulfate is used to treat eclampsia. Choice **c** is incorrect. Oral and epidural medications such as Stadol and Nubain are used for management of labor pain but prostaglandin E is not.

Category: Physiological Integrity: Pharmacology

Subcategory: Maternal Infant: Medication Administration

138. c. The nurse recognizes the proper administration of an enema involves: placing the client in the Sims', or a knee to chest, position; encouraging the client to retain the solution for at least 5 minutes to promote the effectiveness of the enema; and washing hands and gloving to decrease the transmission of microorganisms. The nurse should compress the container to release the solution under positive pressure verses gravity. The solution should be warm, not chilled. The nurse should insert the enema into the full length of the rectum.

Category: Physiological Integrity: Basic Care and Comfort

Subcategory: Medical Surgical: Gastrointestinal Disorders

139. b. Xanax is used to treat anxiety. Choice **a** is incorrect. Disulfiram (Antabuse) is used to treat alcohol abuse. Choice **c** is incorrect. To treat delirium, the underlying cause must first be determined and treated. Choice **d** is incorrect. Medications used to treat depression include barbiturates, sedatives, monoamine oxidase inhibitors, selective serotonin reuptake inhibitors, and tricyclic antidepressants.

Category: Physiological Integrity: Pharmacology

Subcategory: Mental Health: Medication Administration

140. d. The feeding should be placed on hold prior to placing the client in the supine position during the bed bath. The feeding should then be resumed once the bath is completed and the head of the bed elevated. Choice **a** is incorrect. Checking for tube placement is important but the feeding should be placed on hold prior to the head of the bed being lowered to prevent aspiration. Choice **b** is incorrect. Decreasing the feeding tube rate to 20 cc per hour will not prevent the client from aspirating when placed in the supine position. The feeding should be placed on hold to prevent aspiration. Choice **c** is incorrect. It is not necessary to disconnect the feeding tube when the client is placed in the supine position. The feeding should be placed on hold and then resumed once the bath is completed and the head of the bed elevated.
Category: Safe and Effective Care Environment: Coordinated Care
Subcategory: Adult: Gastrointestinal

141. b. Utilizing heel lifts, also commonly referred to as "bunny boots," "heel boots," and "heel lift boots," will off-load pressure from the client's heels. Choice **a** is incorrect. When utilizing a pillow to remove pressure from the client's heels, the pillow should be positioned under the legs with the heels dangling off the pillow's edge so that they are not touching the mattress or pillow surface. Choice **c** is incorrect. Placing the client in a supine position will continue to place pressure on the client's heels unless the heels are positioned correctly using a pillow, blanket, or heel lifts. Choice **d** is incorrect. Positioning the client into the high-Fowler's position—with the patient sitting straight up at a 90 degree angle—will continue to place pressure on the client's heels unless the heels are positioned correctly using a pillow, blanket, or heel lifts.
Category: Safe and Effective Care Environment: Coordinated Care
Subcategory: Adult: Integumentary

142. The correct answer is *HIPAA or Health Insurance Portability and Accountability Act.* The Health Insurance Portability and Accountability Act was designed to protect clients' personal health information (PHI). Discussing a client's test results in a public place where the conversation can be overheard by others is considered a HIPAA violation because the client's PHI is disclosed without the client's consent.
Category: Safe and Effective Care Environment: Coordinated Care
Subcategory: Adult: Miscellaneous

143. c. Antacids decrease gastric acidity and should be continued even if the client's symptoms subside. Choice **a** is incorrect. If the client develops cardiovascular problems, the client should avoid antacids containing sodium, not magnesium. Choice **b** is incorrect. Antacids should be taken 1 to 2 hours before meals. Choice **d** is incorrect. Because other medications may interfere with antacid action, the client should avoid taking antacids concomitantly with other prescribed medications.

Category: Physiological Integrity: Pharmacology

Subcategory: Gastrointestinal Disorders

144. b. It is recommended that an ostomy pouch be emptied when it is $\frac{1}{3}$ to $\frac{1}{2}$ full to prevent the weight of the effluent from pulling the pouch away from the skin, causing leaks. Since **b** is correct, additional teaching is not needed. Choice **a** is incorrect. While the nurse may choose to empty the pouch when it is $\frac{1}{4}$ full, it is not necessary. Choice **c** is incorrect. Waiting until the pouch is $\frac{3}{4}$ full before it is emptied may cause the weight of the effluent to cause the pouch to pull away from the skin, causing leakage. Choice **d** is incorrect. Waiting until the pouch is $\frac{7}{8}$ full before it is emptied may cause the weight of the effluent to cause the pouch to pull away from the skin, causing leakage.

Category: Safe and Effective Care Environment: Coordinated Care

Subcategory: Adult: Gastrointestinal

145. b. When it is possible, the recipient site should be elevated to prevent edema formation. Choice **a** is incorrect. The nurse should not change the dressing twice daily. The dressing is commonly left in place until the physician transcribes an order to have the dressing changed. Choice **c** is incorrect. The client should not complete range-of-motion exercises on the recipient site; this could cause the graft to separate from the surrounding skin. Choice **d** is incorrect. The site should not be left open to air. Often the nurse is ordered to apply a warm sterile compress to the recipient site.

Category: Physiological Integrity: Physiological Adaptation

Subcategory: Integumentary Disorders

146. c. An INR between 2 and 3 is considered therapeutic for a client on Coumadin. Since **c** is correct, additional teaching is not needed. Choice **a** is incorrect. An INR between 0 and 1 is subtherapeutic for a client on Coumadin. Choice **b** is incorrect. An INR between 1 and 2 is subtherapeutic for a client on Coumadin. Choice **d** is incorrect. An INR between 3 and 4 is considered too high for a client on Coumadin.

Category: Safe and Effective Care Environment: Coordinated Care

Subcategory: Adult: Hematopoietic System

147. a. Occupational therapists focus on fine motor movement. Choice **b** is incorrect. Physical therapists focus on strength and gross motor movement. Choice **c** is incorrect. Recreational therapists focus on the use of sports, games, crafts, and music to help rebuild clients' confidence and resume their lives after injury and/or disability. Choice **d** is incorrect. Speech therapists evaluate, diagnose, treat, and prevent speech, language, cognitive-communicative, and swallowing disorders.

Category: Safe and Effective Care Environment: Coordinated Care

Subcategory: Adult: Musculoskeletal

148. c. Scoliosis is the lateral curvature of the spine and findings include: unequal shoulder heights, prominent scapula, curved spinal column, and asymmetry of the back. Choice **a** is incorrect. Dowager's hump presents as a hump across the upper back. It is more correctly referred to as kyphosis. Choice **b** is incorrect. Kyphosis presents with the appearance of poor posture and a hump on the upper back. It is also referred to as a dowager's hump. Choice **d** is incorrect. While uneven leg length would cause one hip to be higher than the other, it would not cause the prominent scapula and curvature of the spine shown on the picture.

Category: Physiological Integrity: Physiological Adaptation

Subcategory: Pediatric: Musculoskeletal

149. c. Orthopnea is a symptom of left-sided heart failure. Choice **a** is incorrect. Hepatomegaly is a symptom of right-sided heart failure. Choice **b** is incorrect. Jugular vein distension is a symptom of right-sided heart failure. Choice **d** is incorrect. Right upper quadrant pain is a symptom of right-sided heart failure.

Category: Safe and Effective Care Environment: Coordinated Care

Subcategory: Adult: Cardiovascular

150. c. A client with an irrational belief of love from a person with higher social status is experiencing an erotomania subtype delusional disorder. Choice **a** is incorrect. Clients with an irrational belief of their bodies not functioning correctly or being disfigured are experiencing a somatic subtype of delusional disorder. Choice **b** is incorrect. Clients with an irrational belief of a conspiracy against them are experiencing a persecutory subtype of delusional disorder. Choice **d** is incorrect. A client with an irrational belief of unfaithfulness from his or her significant other has jealous subtype delusional disorder.

Category: Physiological Integrity: Physiological Adaptation

Subcategory: Mental Health: Delusional Disorders

151. d. Diabetes insipidus (DI) is a disorder characterized by intense thirst and the excretion of large amounts of urine. It commonly results from the body's inability to produce, store, or release a key hormone, but DI can also occur when the kidneys are unable to respond properly to that hormone. Vasopressin is given subcutaneously in the acute management of DI. Choice **a** is incorrect. Furosemide is utilized to produce diuresis and is contraindicated in this situation. Choice **b** is incorrect. If the client were experiencing diabetes mellitus, the nurse would administer insulin. Choice **c** is incorrect. Potassium chloride is indicated for hypokalemia and is not required in this situation.

Category: Physiological Integrity: Pharmacology

Subcategory: Endocrine Disorders

152. c. Increased protein in the diet can promote wound healing. Choice **a** is incorrect. Decreased fat intake is recommended for clients with cardiovascular disease and obesity. Choice **b** is incorrect. Decreased sodium intake is recommended for clients with cardiovascular disease. Choice **d** is incorrect. The client should be instructed to increase protein, not carbohydrates, to promote wound healing.

Category: Safe and Effective Care Environment: Coordination of Care

Subcategory: Adult: Integumentary

153. b. The nurse should let the physician know that the client has changed her mind and no longer wants the debridement. Choice **a** is incorrect. The nurse does not know whether everything will be okay. The client has the right to refuse the treatment. Choice **c** is incorrect. The client has the right to refuse the treatment. This statement implies to the client that he or she does not have the right to refuse treatment. Choice **d** is incorrect. While a debridement is a common procedure, this statement does not respect the client's decision to refuse the treatment.

Category: Safe and Effective Care Environment: Coordinated Care

Subcategory: Adult: Integumentary

154. b. Trauma is not a contraindication for organs not affected by organ donation. Therefore, more staff training on organ donation is necessary. Choice **a** is incorrect. While age restrictions vary by organ being donated, most require the client's age to be less than 65. Choice **c** is incorrect. Malignancy is a contraindication to organ donation. Choice **d** is incorrect. Communicable diseases are a contraindication to organ donation.

Category: Safe and Effective Care Environment: Coordinated Care

Subcategory: Adult: Death and Dying

155. a. The nurse should always wash his or her hands before entering a client's room. Additionally, a client with a MRSA infection should be placed in contact precautions, which include gowning and gloving prior to patient contact. Choice **b** is incorrect. While a client with a MRSA infection should be placed in contact precautions, which includes utilization of a gown and gloves for patient care, a mask is not required. Choices **c** and **d** are incorrect. The nurse should wash his or her hands prior to entering any client room. The client with a MRSA infection should be placed on contact precautions, which necessitate the use of a gown and gloves, but a mask is not required.
Category: Safe and Effective Care Environment: Safety and Infection Control
Subcategory: Adult: Infectious Diseases

156. a. By asking what the voices are saying to the client, the nurse can assess whether the client is at risk of harming himself or others. Choice **b** is incorrect. While moving the client to a room by the nursing station allows for closer observation of the client, it does not allow the nurse to assess the client's risk for harming him- or herself or others. Choice **c** is incorrect. Contacting the registered nurse will not facilitate the determination of whether the client is at risk for harming him- or herself or others. Choice **d** is incorrect. By telling the client that no one else is in the room, the nurse sets the stage for conflict regarding the voices and does not facilitate the determination of whether the client is at risk for harming him- or herself or others.
Category: Physiological Integrity: Reduction of Risk Potential
Subcategory: Mental Health: Schizophrenia Disorders

157. d. Due to the potential side effects of sedation, dizziness, and confusion, the best time for the client to take the medication is prior to going to bed. Choices **a**, **b**, and **c** are incorrect. While the client could take the medication at breakfast, lunch, or dinner, the best time is before bed due to the potential side effects of sedation, dizziness, and confusion.
Category: Safe and Effective Care Environment: Safety and Infection Control
Subcategory: Adult: Neurological

158. b. The nurse should initially give two breaths followed by chest compressions. Choice **a** is incorrect. The nurse should initially give the client two breaths, not five chest compressions. Choice **c** is incorrect. The nurse should stay with the client and not leave the room. The other staff members can/will bring the code/emergency cart to the client's room. Choice **d** is incorrect. It is not within the LPN's scope of practice to defibrillate the client.
Category: Physiological Integrity: Physiological Adaptation
Subcategory: Cardiovascular Disorders

159. a. The nurse should assess for the pedal pulse with a Doppler. Choice **b** is incorrect. While the capillary refill does provide some information relating to blood flow to the extremity, using a Doppler to assess the pulse provides the nurse with definitive information relating to blood flow within the extremity. Choice **c** is incorrect. The nurse should first determine whether the pedal pulse can be heard with the Doppler. If the pulse is not audible with the Doppler, the nurse should then contact the physician. Choice **d** is incorrect. The client has decreased arterial blood flow to the extremity. Elevating the extremity will further decrease the blood flow.
Category: Safe and Effective Care Environment: Safety and Infection Control
Subcategory: Adult: Peripheral Vascular Disorder

160. b. The medication should be given with food or at mealtime. Food protects the stomach from becoming upset. Choice **a** is incorrect. Giving the medication at bedtime will not necessarily reduce the gastrointestinal side effects. Choice **c** is incorrect. Administering the medication with an antacid will not necessarily reduce the gastrointestinal side effects. Choice **d** is incorrect. Drinking an increased amount of fluids will not necessarily reduce the gastrointestinal side effects.
Category: Physiological Integrity: Pharmacology
Subcategory: Respiratory Disorders

161. a. Use of a bed/chair alarm will alert the staff when the client gets out of the bed/chair so that they can ensure that the client does not wander out of the room. Choice **b** is incorrect. A lowboy bed can prevent the client from harm due to a fall but will not prevent the client from wandering from the room. Choice **c** is incorrect. A vest requires a physician's order and there is no indication that this client is in need of being restrained. Choice **d** is incorrect. Wrist restraints require a physician's order. There is no indication that this client is need of wrist restraints at this time.
Category: Safe and Effective Care Environment: Safety and Infection Control
Subcategory: Adult: Neurological

162. c. Clients receiving systemic radiation are at risk for leukopenia (decreased white blood count) and thrombocytopenia (decreased platelets). Choice **a** is incorrect. Clients receiving systemic radiation are at risk for leukopenia (decreased white blood count) but dysgeusia (decreased sense of taste) occurs with localized radiation to the head and neck. Choice **b** is incorrect. Clients receiving systemic radiation are at risk for thrombocytopenia (decreased platelets) but dysgeusia (decreased sense of taste) occurs with localized radiation to the head and neck. Choice **d** is incorrect. Clients receiving systemic radiation are at risk for leukopenia (decreased white blood count) but xerostomia (dry mouth) occurs with localized radiation to the head and neck.
Category: Safe and Effective Care Environment: Safety and Infection Control
Subcategory: Adult: Cancer

163. b. The client should be repositioned every 1 to 2 hours to prevent the occurrence of a hospital-acquired pressure ulcer. Choice **a** is incorrect. While repositioning the client every 30 minutes will help to prevent pressure ulcer formation, this schedule may be difficult to maintain. Standards of care indicate that the client should be repositioned every 1 to 2 hours. Choices **c** and **d** are incorrect. Standards of care indicate that the client should be repositioned every 1 to 2 hours to prevent hospital-acquired pressure ulcer formation.
Category: Safe and Effective Care Environment: Safety and Infection Control
Subcategory: Adult: Integumentary

164. d. The nurse should utilize the gloves, gown, and mask when taking the blood pressure of a client on droplet precautions. Choice **a** is incorrect. When the nurse is taking the blood pressure of a client on droplet precautions, the nurse should utilize gloves and a gown but does not need to utilize goggles. Choice **b** is incorrect. The nurse should utilize a gown and mask but does not need to utilize the goggles when taking the blood pressure of a client on droplet precautions. Choice **c** is incorrect. The nurse should utilize gloves and a mask when taking the blood pressure of a client on droplet precautions but does not need to utilize goggles.
Category: Safe and Effective Care Environment: Safety and Infection Control
Subcategory: Adult: Infectious Disease

165. b. Women who experience their first period after the age of 12 do not have an increased risk for breast cancer. Choice **a** is incorrect. Women who experience their first pregnancy after the age of 35 have an increased risk for breast cancer. Choice **c** is incorrect. Women with high breast-density have an increased risk for breast cancer. Choice **d** is incorrect. Women who experience postmenopausal weight gain have an increased risk for breast cancer.
Category: Health Promotion and Maintenance
Subcategory: Adult: Cancer

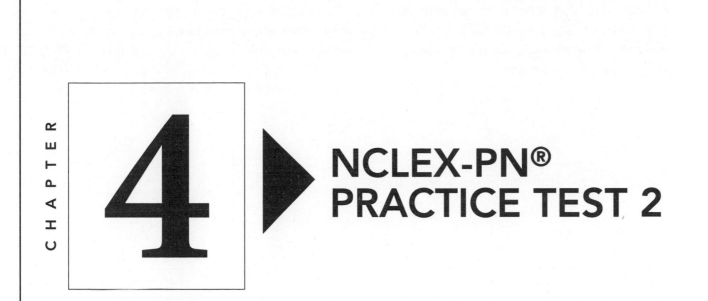

4 ▶ NCLEX-PN®
PRACTICE TEST 2

This examination has been designed to test your understanding of the content included on the National Council Licensure Examination for Licensed Practical/Vocational Nurses (NCLEX-PN®). Becoming comfortable with the examination format and logistics will help you be more relaxed when it comes to actually sitting for the test, enabling you to perform at your best.

The actual NCLEX-PN® exam is computer adaptive, which means all examinees will have a different number of test questions depending on how many and what types of questions they answer correctly and how many they answer incorrectly. All test takers must answer a minimum of 85 items, and the maximum number of items that the candidate may answer is 205 during the allotted five-hour time period. This LearningExpress practice exam has 165 questions, and you should allow yourself four hours to complete it.

After you have completed the exam, look at the answer key to read the rationale for both the correct and incorrect choices, as well as the sources of the information. It is recommended that you utilize the sources to thoroughly review information that was problematic for you. Because the NCLEX-PN® examination is graded on a sliding scale that is based on the difficulty of each particular exam, we are unable to predict how many correct answers would equate to an actual passing grade on this practice exam.

Completion of this examination represents the culmination of extensive test preparation. You have worked very hard to review the information from your NCLEX-PN® curriculum, and now it is your time to shine. Good luck!

Practice Test 2 Answer Sheet

1.	ⓐ ⓑ ⓒ ⓓ	56.	ⓐ ⓑ ⓒ ⓓ	111.	ⓐ ⓑ ⓒ ⓓ
2.	ⓐ ⓑ ⓒ ⓓ	57.	ⓐ ⓑ ⓒ ⓓ	112.	ⓐ ⓑ ⓒ ⓓ
3.	_____	58.	ⓐ ⓑ ⓒ ⓓ	113.	ⓐ ⓑ ⓒ ⓓ
4.	ⓐ ⓑ ⓒ ⓓ	59.	_____	114.	ⓐ ⓑ ⓒ ⓓ
5.	ⓐ ⓑ ⓒ ⓓ	60.	ⓐ ⓑ ⓒ ⓓ	115.	ⓐ ⓑ ⓒ ⓓ
6.	ⓐ ⓑ ⓒ ⓓ	61.	ⓐ ⓑ ⓒ ⓓ	116.	ⓐ ⓑ ⓒ ⓓ
7.	ⓐ ⓑ ⓒ ⓓ	62.	ⓐ ⓑ ⓒ ⓓ	117.	ⓐ ⓑ ⓒ ⓓ
8.	ⓐ ⓑ ⓒ ⓓ	63.	ⓐ ⓑ ⓒ ⓓ	118.	ⓐ ⓑ ⓒ ⓓ
9.	ⓐ ⓑ ⓒ ⓓ	64.	ⓐ ⓑ ⓒ ⓓ	119.	ⓐ ⓑ ⓒ ⓓ
10.	ⓐ ⓑ ⓒ ⓓ	65.	ⓐ ⓑ ⓒ ⓓ	120.	ⓐ ⓑ ⓒ ⓓ
11.	ⓐ ⓑ ⓒ ⓓ	66.	ⓐ ⓑ ⓒ ⓓ	121.	ⓐ ⓑ ⓒ ⓓ
12.	ⓐ ⓑ ⓒ ⓓ	67.	ⓐ ⓑ ⓒ ⓓ	122.	ⓐ ⓑ ⓒ ⓓ
13.	_____	68.	ⓐ ⓑ ⓒ ⓓ	123.	ⓐ ⓑ ⓒ ⓓ
14.	ⓐ ⓑ ⓒ ⓓ	69.	ⓐ ⓑ ⓒ ⓓ	124.	ⓐ ⓑ ⓒ ⓓ
15.	ⓐ ⓑ ⓒ ⓓ	70.	ⓐ ⓑ ⓒ ⓓ	125.	ⓐ ⓑ ⓒ ⓓ
16.	ⓐ ⓑ ⓒ ⓓ	71.	ⓐ ⓑ ⓒ ⓓ	126.	ⓐ ⓑ ⓒ ⓓ
17.	_____	72.	ⓐ ⓑ ⓒ ⓓ	127.	ⓐ ⓑ ⓒ ⓓ
18.	ⓐ ⓑ ⓒ ⓓ	73.	ⓐ ⓑ ⓒ ⓓ	128.	ⓐ ⓑ ⓒ ⓓ
19.	ⓐ ⓑ ⓒ ⓓ	74.	ⓐ ⓑ ⓒ ⓓ	129.	ⓐ ⓑ ⓒ ⓓ
20.	ⓐ ⓑ ⓒ ⓓ	75.	ⓐ ⓑ ⓒ ⓓ	130.	ⓐ ⓑ ⓒ ⓓ
21.	_____	76.	ⓐ ⓑ ⓒ ⓓ	131.	ⓐ ⓑ ⓒ ⓓ
22.	ⓐ ⓑ ⓒ ⓓ	77.	ⓐ ⓑ ⓒ ⓓ	132.	ⓐ ⓑ ⓒ ⓓ
23.	ⓐ ⓑ ⓒ ⓓ	78.	ⓐ ⓑ ⓒ ⓓ	133.	ⓐ ⓑ ⓒ ⓓ
24.	ⓐ ⓑ ⓒ ⓓ	79.	ⓐ ⓑ ⓒ ⓓ	134.	ⓐ ⓑ ⓒ ⓓ
25.	ⓐ ⓑ ⓒ ⓓ	80.	ⓐ ⓑ ⓒ ⓓ	135.	ⓐ ⓑ ⓒ ⓓ
26.	ⓐ ⓑ ⓒ ⓓ	81.	_____	136.	ⓐ ⓑ ⓒ ⓓ
27.	_____	82.	ⓐ ⓑ ⓒ ⓓ	137.	ⓐ ⓑ ⓒ ⓓ
28.	ⓐ ⓑ ⓒ ⓓ	83.	ⓐ ⓑ ⓒ ⓓ	138.	ⓐ ⓑ ⓒ ⓓ
29.	ⓐ ⓑ ⓒ ⓓ	84.	ⓐ ⓑ ⓒ ⓓ	139.	ⓐ ⓑ ⓒ ⓓ
30.	ⓐ ⓑ ⓒ ⓓ	85.	ⓐ ⓑ ⓒ ⓓ	140.	ⓐ ⓑ ⓒ ⓓ
31.	ⓐ ⓑ ⓒ ⓓ	86.	ⓐ ⓑ ⓒ ⓓ	141.	ⓐ ⓑ ⓒ ⓓ
32.	_____	87.	ⓐ ⓑ ⓒ ⓓ	142.	ⓐ ⓑ ⓒ ⓓ
33.	ⓐ ⓑ ⓒ ⓓ	88.	ⓐ ⓑ ⓒ ⓓ	143.	ⓐ ⓑ ⓒ ⓓ
34.	_____	89.	ⓐ ⓑ ⓒ ⓓ	144.	ⓐ ⓑ ⓒ ⓓ
35.	ⓐ ⓑ ⓒ ⓓ	90.	ⓐ ⓑ ⓒ ⓓ	145.	ⓐ ⓑ ⓒ ⓓ
36.	ⓐ ⓑ ⓒ ⓓ	91.	ⓐ ⓑ ⓒ ⓓ	146.	ⓐ ⓑ ⓒ ⓓ
37.	ⓐ ⓑ ⓒ ⓓ	92.	ⓐ ⓑ ⓒ ⓓ	147.	ⓐ ⓑ ⓒ ⓓ
38.	ⓐ ⓑ ⓒ ⓓ	93.	ⓐ ⓑ ⓒ ⓓ	148.	ⓐ ⓑ ⓒ ⓓ
39.	ⓐ ⓑ ⓒ ⓓ	94.	ⓐ ⓑ ⓒ ⓓ	149.	ⓐ ⓑ ⓒ ⓓ
40.	ⓐ ⓑ ⓒ ⓓ	95.	ⓐ ⓑ ⓒ ⓓ	150.	ⓐ ⓑ ⓒ ⓓ
41.	ⓐ ⓑ ⓒ ⓓ	96.	ⓐ ⓑ ⓒ ⓓ	151.	ⓐ ⓑ ⓒ ⓓ
42.	ⓐ ⓑ ⓒ ⓓ	97.	ⓐ ⓑ ⓒ ⓓ	152.	ⓐ ⓑ ⓒ ⓓ
43.	ⓐ ⓑ ⓒ ⓓ	98.	ⓐ ⓑ ⓒ ⓓ	153.	ⓐ ⓑ ⓒ ⓓ
44.	ⓐ ⓑ ⓒ ⓓ	99.	ⓐ ⓑ ⓒ ⓓ	154.	ⓐ ⓑ ⓒ ⓓ
45.	ⓐ ⓑ ⓒ ⓓ	100.	ⓐ ⓑ ⓒ ⓓ	155.	ⓐ ⓑ ⓒ ⓓ
46.	ⓐ ⓑ ⓒ ⓓ	101.	ⓐ ⓑ ⓒ ⓓ	156.	_____
47.	ⓐ ⓑ ⓒ ⓓ	102.	ⓐ ⓑ ⓒ ⓓ	157.	ⓐ ⓑ ⓒ ⓓ
48.	ⓐ ⓑ ⓒ ⓓ	103.	ⓐ ⓑ ⓒ ⓓ	158.	ⓐ ⓑ ⓒ ⓓ
49.	ⓐ ⓑ ⓒ ⓓ	104.	ⓐ ⓑ ⓒ ⓓ	159.	ⓐ ⓑ ⓒ ⓓ
50.	_____	105.	ⓐ ⓑ ⓒ ⓓ	160.	ⓐ ⓑ ⓒ ⓓ
51.	ⓐ ⓑ ⓒ ⓓ	106.	ⓐ ⓑ ⓒ ⓓ	161.	ⓐ ⓑ ⓒ ⓓ
52.	ⓐ ⓑ ⓒ ⓓ	107.	ⓐ ⓑ ⓒ ⓓ	162.	_____
53.	ⓐ ⓑ ⓒ ⓓ	108.	_____	153.	ⓐ ⓑ ⓒ ⓓ
54.	ⓐ ⓑ ⓒ ⓓ	109.	ⓐ ⓑ ⓒ ⓓ	164.	ⓐ ⓑ ⓒ ⓓ
55.	ⓐ ⓑ ⓒ ⓓ	110.	ⓐ ⓑ ⓒ ⓓ	165.	ⓐ ⓑ ⓒ ⓓ

Questions

1. The nurse is participating in the care of a male client on an orthopedic nursing unit. The client is ordered continuous passive motion (CPM). Which of the following statements if made by the nurse indicates the need for further teaching?
   a. "The client receives physical therapy so there is no need for CPM."
   b. "The use of CPM helps to prevent the development of adhesions."
   c. "I will monitor the client's skin while the CPM device is in use."
   d. "I will observe for bleeding when the client receives CPM."

2. The nurse is participating in the care of a client with end-stage renal failure. The physician orders a palliative care consult because the client wishes no further medical interventions. Which of the following should the nurse anticipate based on her knowledge of palliative care?
   a. decreasing pain medication administration
   b. decreasing the amount of supplemental oxygen
   c. increasing oral and intravenous fluid amounts
   d. increasing the administration of antianxiety medications

3. The nurse is assisting in the care of a pregnant client whose last menstrual period was September 15, 2012. Using Nacgele's rule, the client's due date is _____.

4. The nurse is working in a pediatrician's office. A mother who recently separated from her husband states that she is worried because her 6-year-old boy started to wet the bed again. The nurse knows that the boy is most likely experiencing which of the following?
   a. passive aggression
   b. regression
   c. repression
   d. suppression

5. The nurse is reinforcing teaching for a diabetic client who must mix regular insulin and NPH insulin in the same syringe. Which of the following actions, if performed by the client, indicates the need for further instruction?
   a. injecting air into the NPH vial first
   b. injecting an amount of air equal to the prescribed dosage of insulin into the vial
   c. withdrawing the NPH insulin first
   d. withdrawing the regular insulin first

6. The nurse is participating in the care of a client on a cardiac telemetry unit. While completing morning care, the nurse notes the following ECG rhythm on the monitor.

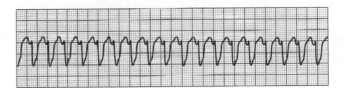

   The nurse correctly identifies this as which of the following?
   a. atrial fibrillation
   b. atrial flutter
   c. ventricular fibrillation
   d. ventricular tachycardia

7. A nurse is assisting in a community education program on fetal development. The nurse knows that no additional teaching is needed when a participant comments that the fetal heartbeat can be heard with a Doppler at which time during the pregnancy?

   a. 6 to 8 weeks

   b. 8 to 10 weeks

   c. 10 to 12 weeks

   d. 12 to 14 weeks

8. The nurse is caring for a client who is ordered droplet precautions. Which protective equipment would the nurse utilize when caring for this client?

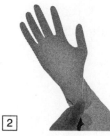

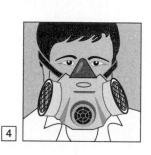

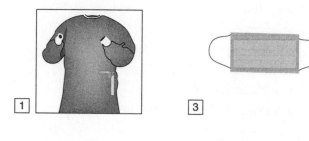

   a. 1

   b. 2

   c. 3

   d. 4

9. A client begins to cry after hearing that her cancer is inoperable. The nurse hands the client a tissue and responds appropriately with which of the following?

   a. "Everything will be okay."

   b. "I will stay here with you."

   c. "My father had the same cancer."

   d. "You need a second opinion."

10. The nurse has just completed administering a client's morning dosage of NPH insulin. The client asks the nurse, "If my blood sugar is going to drop, when will it occur?" Which of the following is the nurse's best response?

   a. 2 to 4 hours after the administration of the insulin

   b. 4 to 12 hours after the administration of the insulin

   c. 16 to 18 hours after the administration of the insulin

   d. 18 to 24 hours after the administration of the insulin

11. The nurse is communicating with an adolescent regarding sexual activity. Which of the following phrases should the nurse AVOID to foster therapeutic communication?

   a. "Are you saying . . ."

   b. "It sounds as if . . ."

   c. "Tell me . . ."

   d. "You should . . ."

12. The nurse is caring for a client who is ordered Zofran (ondansetron) as needed. The nurse recognizes this medication is administered for which of the following?

   a. gastrointestinal irritation

   b. incisional pain

   c. nausea and vomiting

   d. urinary retention

13. The nurse is assisting in the planning of care for an 18-month-old boy. The nurse demonstrates an understanding of Erickson's Theory of Psychosocial Development when care is planned for a child in the stage of

   _____.

14. The nurse is participating in the care of a client on a telemetry step-down unit who is prescribed digoxin (Lanoxin). The physician has ordered a digoxin level to rule out toxicity. The nurse understands that which of the following is a therapeutic serum level/range for digoxin?
a. 3.5 to 5.5 ng/mL
b. 3 to 5 ng/mL
c. 1.2 to 2.8 ng/mL
d. 0.5 to 2 ng/mL

15. The medical-surgical floor where the nurse works is very busy with a high admission and discharge rate. The floor has been short-staffed for the past month due to two nurses quitting. The nurse has worked many overtime/additional shifts. Which of the following are signs that the nurse may be starting to experience burnout?
a. empathy
b. hyperactivity
c. irritability
d. optimism

16. A nurse is assisting in the plan of care for a client with an anxiety disorder. The plan should incorporate care for a client whose physiological symptoms include all EXCEPT which of the following?
a. decreased urinary output
b. elevated blood pressure
c. shallow respirations
d. tremors

17. The nurse must administer 6,000 units of heparin subcutaneously. The vial reads 10,000 units/mL. How many milliliters of heparin should the nurse draw up in the syringe?

_____

18. The nurse is assisting in the assessment of a pregnant woman who is 38 years old. The nurse knows that this woman is at risk for which of the following?
a. anemia
b. hyperemesis gravidarum
c. placenta previa
d. post-term delivery

19. The nurse is caring for a client complaining of constipation. The nurse is preparing to administer the client's PRN dosage of milk of magnesia. The order reads two teaspoons by mouth. How many milliliters will the nurse administer?
a. 2
b. 5
c. 10
d. 15

20. The LPN is participating in the care of a postoperative client. Which of the following is the best intervention to aid in preventing postoperative complications?
a. bladder and bowel monitoring
b. early ambulation
c. pain management
d. progressive diet

21. The nurse is documenting the height of a 14-year-old boy in centimeters. The boy measures 58 inches tall. The nurse documents the boy's height as _____ cm.

22. The LPN is participating in the care of a client complaining of nausea, right lower abdominal pain, and a fever of 101 degrees F. Which of the following will the nurse expect to be completed first?
    a. an abdominal X-ray
    b. administration of a soap-suds enema
    c. blood draw for CBC (complete blood count)
    d. deep palpation of the right abdominal quadrant

23. A nurse is viewing the chart of a client at a mental health clinic. The client is documented as having agoraphobia. The nurse expects to care for a client who is afraid of which of the following?
    a. crowds
    b. death
    c. heights
    d. water

24. A pregnant client comes to the outpatient clinic due to having a positive home pregnancy test. The nurse knows that home pregnancy tests are based on the presence of which of the following hormones in the urine?
    a. maternal estrogen-progesterone
    b. human chorionic gonadotropin
    c. follicle-stimulating hormone
    d. alpha-fetoprotien

25. The LPN is participating in the care of a male client who experienced a myocardial infarction (MI) seven weeks ago. The client has just completed an outpatient cardiac rehabilitation session. The client asks the nurse: "Is it safe for me to have sex yet?" The nurse's response should include which of the following information?
    a. "It is recommended that erectile dysfunction medication and nitroglycerin are taken prior to sexual relations."
    b. "Resting several hours prior to having intercourse would be helpful."
    c. "Sexual intercourse should be avoided for five months after an MI."
    d. "Taking nitroglycerin as prescribed prior to sexual intercourse can be helpful."

26. The nurse is caring for a 60-year-old client being seen in the physician's office. The client is diagnosed with pernicious anemia. Which comment, if made by the client, offers the nurse the most concern related to this diagnosis?
    a. "I had trouble reading the newspaper over the last month."
    b. "I've started having pain in my legs."
    c. "My knees hurt when I walk up and down stairs."
    d. "My headaches are getting worse."

27. The nurse needs to administer 0.2 grams of Dilantin (phenytoin) orally to a client diagnosed with a seizure disorder. The medication label states 100 mg capsules. The nurse prepares how many capsule(s) to administer to the client?

    _____

28. The nurse is preparing to collect a sputum culture from a female client. The nurse should plan to complete which of the following?
   a. Collect a sample every time the client has a productive cough.
   b. Collect the sputum sample during the early morning hours.
   c. Instruct the client to rinse her mouth with mouthwash prior to obtaining the sample.
   d. Tell the client to increase fluid intake prior to sample collection.

29. The nurse is participating in the care of a client who is scheduled for a laryngectomy. When preparing the client for surgery, which of the following is essential for the nurse to complete?
   a. assessing whether the client can read and write and at what level
   b. ensuring the client has learned how to read lips
   c. reinforcing the esophageal speech teaching that was completed
   d. telling the client a sore throat will follow the surgery

30. A male client in a mental health facility begins to yell at the nurse when visiting hours are over and the client's visitor leaves. The nurse should
   a. avoid the client until he calms down.
   b. talk with client about his anger.
   c. tell the visitor to come earlier next time.
   d. tell the client to go to his room.

31. The nurse is caring for a female client who is scheduled for a bronchoscopy the following day. The nurse will plan to
   a. administer a cleansing enema the evening prior to the procedure.
   b. increase the client's fluid intake prior to the procedure.
   c. instruct the client that she will be NPO after midnight.
   d. withhold the client's medications prior to the procedure.

32. The nurse is participating in the care of a client receiving continuous bladder irrigation following prostate surgery. The client received 1,700 mL of normal saline irrigating solution and the output in the client's urine drainage bag is 2,600 mL at the end of the nursing shift. How many milliliters of urine will the nurse record as output for the shift?

_____

33. The nurse is working at an outpatient clinic when she is asked to make an appointment for a client to have an amniocentesis. The nurse knows that the amniocentesis will detect which of the following fetal complications?
   a. cystic fibrosis
   b. fetal alcohol syndrome
   c. meconium aspiration
   d. neural tube defects

34. The nurse is caring for a client at risk for developing hypocalcemia due to a recent thyroidectomy. The nurse recognizes that which of the following are signs and symptoms of hypocalcemia? Select all that apply.

1. aphasia
2. Chvostek's sign
3. numbness
4. paresthesias
5. polyuria
6. seizures

35. The nurse is caring for an adolescent after tonsil surgery who is ordered E-mycin (erythromycin) 750 mg po t.i.d. Available is E-mycin suspension 250 mg per 10 mLs. How many teaspoons should the nurse give to the adolescent?
a. 2
b. 4
c. 6
d. 8

36. The nurse is caring for a client with a urinary catheter. The physician has ordered irrigation of the catheter. The physician's order did not specify the type of solution that was to be used. Which of the following solutions is most appropriate for the nurse to use for the procedure?
a. distilled water
b. diluted hydrogen peroxide
c. room-temperature tap water
d. sterile normal saline solution

37. The nurse is caring for a client on a medical-surgical unit who is diagnosed with obstructive jaundice. The nurse recognizes that signs and symptoms of obstructive jaundice include which of the following?
a. dark brown urine
b. green, watery stool
c. red, dry skin
d. tan, thick sputum

38. The nurse is participating in the care of a client with expressive aphasia as a result of a cerebral vascular accident (CVA). Utilizing the image shown here, identify what area of the brain was affected by the stroke.

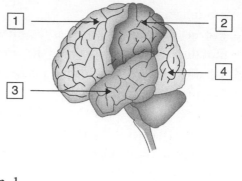

a. 1
b. 2
c. 3
d. 4

39. A nursing assistant informs the nurse that she is concerned because a woman who has just given birth has bloody discharge. The nurse explains that this is most likely a sign that the woman is experiencing
a. hemorrhage.
b. lochia rubra.
c. uterine subinvolution.
d. uterine infection.

40. The nurse is caring for a client experiencing an overdose of an opioid. The nurse anticipates an order for which of the following?
a. activated charcoal
b. antabuse
c. Narcan
d. vitamin K

41. The nurse is caring for a client diagnosed with allergic asthma. The client is prescribed an Intal (cromolyn sodium) inhaler. The nurse understands a common side effect of this medication is which of the following?

   a. bronchospasms
   b. constipation
   c. diarrhea
   d. insomnia

42. The nurse is caring for a male client with the chest appearance depicted in the image shown here. The nurse suspects the client has a diagnosis of which of the following?

   a. bronchitis
   b. emphysema
   c. osteomalacia
   d. scoliosis

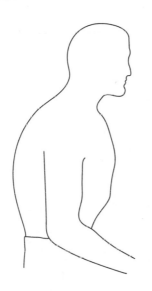

43. The LPN and RN are presenting an educational program to new mothers on breastfeeding. They include the fact that the mothers should try to feed the infant when he or she demonstrates feeding readiness clues. The participants demonstrate understanding when they identify which of the following as such clues? Select all that apply.

   1. hiccups
   2. rooting
   3. waving arms in the air
   4. bringing hand to the mouth

   a. 1 and 2
   b. 2 and 4
   c. 3 and 4
   d. 1 and 4

44. The nurse is assisting in the care of a woman who is 30-hours postdelivery. The woman's uterus is soft and boggy. The nurse's documentation would include a notation related to symptoms of

   a. hemorrhagic shock.
   b. retained placenta.
   c. uterine atony.
   d. uterine inversion.

45. The nurse is participating in the care of a client who has a serum calcium level of 7.8 mg/dL. Given this laboratory value, the nurse will expect to observe which of the following changes on the telemetry tracing?

   a. a prolonged P wave
   b. a prolonged QT interval
   c. a shortened ST segment
   d. a widened T wave

46. The nurse is caring for a client diagnosed with an inner ear disorder. The nurse understands the client is most likely to complain of
    a. burning in the ear.
    b. hearing loss.
    c. pruritus.
    d. tinnitus.

47. The nurse recognizes that which of the following clients is at the greatest risk for developing a fluid volume deficit?
    a. the client with acute renal failure
    b. the client with heart failure
    c. the client with hypertension
    d. the client with an ileostomy

48. A client is taking Vicodin (acetaminophen and hydrocodone) after knee surgery as prescribed and is finding relief from postoperative pain. This client is experiencing which of the following?
    a. dependency
    b. substance use
    c. tolerance
    d. withdrawal

49. A toddler's parents are going through a divorce. The toddler thinks that it is his fault because after a fight with his mother, he once wished that his mother would go away. This is an example of which of the following?
    a. animism
    b. categorization
    c. conservation
    d. magical thinking

50. The nurse is working in a labor and delivery room when the registered nurse states that a woman in labor is experiencing rupture of the uterus. The nurse expects to assist in preparing the woman for _____.

51. The nurse is participating in the care of a client who is retaining carbon dioxide (CO_2) related to respiratory disease. The nurse anticipates that as the client's CO_2 level rises, the client's pH level will
    a. decrease.
    b. double.
    c. increase.
    d. remain unchanged.

52. The nurse is caring for a client the evening following abdominal surgery. The client is ordered "diet as tolerated." The nurse recognizes that which of the following is the most appropriate diet for the client?
    a. clear liquid diet
    b. low-sodium diet
    c. regular diet
    d. soft diet

53. The nurse is caring for a client who is complaining of difficulty having a bowel movement. The nurse understands that which of the following actions best determines whether a client is experiencing a fecal impaction?
    a. assessing the client for diarrhea
    b. auscultating the client's bowel sounds
    c. digitally examining the client's rectum
    d. measuring the client's abdominal girth

54. The nurse is participating in the care of a male client with a chest tube. While the client is being assisted to the bathroom, the chest tube becomes dislodged. The most appropriate initial nursing action when a chest tube is dislodged from the insertion site is to
    a. auscultate the client's breath sounds.
    b. instruct the client to hold his breath.
    c. cover the opening to keep air out.
    d. reinsert the dislodged chest tube.

55. The nurse is assisting in an education program
    for spouses on the symptoms of postpartum
    depression. The nurse instructs the attendees
    on all EXCEPT which of the following?
    a. feelings of competence
    b. feelings of hopelessness
    c. panic attacks
    d. spontaneous outbursts

56. The nurse is caring for a client diagnosed with
    liver failure. The client is jaundiced in appear-
    ance and is complaining of severe itching.
    Which of the following nursing measures is
    most appropriate in decreasing the risk of
    skin breakdown?
    a. applying cornstarch to the client's skin
    b. applying hypoallergenic bed sheets to the
       client's bed
    c. trimming the client's fingernails on a regular
       basis
    d. washing the client with warm water and
       using gentle soap

57. The nurse is caring for a client receiving bex-
    atolol hydrochloride (Betoptic) eye drops for
    glaucoma. The nurse understands that which
    of the following is a common side effect of the
    medication?
    a. decreased blood glucose levels
    b. decreased blood pressure
    c. elevated heart rate
    d. elevated temperature

58. The nurse is caring for a client with an NG
    tube who has been NPO for one week. During
    the nurse's assessment of the client's mouth, no
    saliva is noted, and the client also states dis-
    comfort in the area of the ears. Based on these
    findings, the nurse suspects the client may be
    developing which of the following mouth
    conditions?
    a. parotitis
    b. gingivitis
    c. stomatitis
    d. thrush

59. The nurse is assisting in an educational pro-
    gram for teenagers relating to pregnancy. The
    nurse covers the fact that fertilization occurs
    in the _____.

60. The nurse is participating in the care of a client
    diagnosed with a lower urinary tract infection
    who is being discharged from a medical-
    surgical unit. The client is prescribed Pyridium
    (phenazopyridine hydrochloride) for pain
    relief. The nurse should reinforce which of
    the following?
    a. Discontinue the medication if a headache
       develops.
    b. Expect a reddish-orange discoloration of
       the urine.
    c. Take the medication at bedtime.
    d. Take the medication prior to meals.

61. The nurse is participating in the care of a client
    after a cholecystectomy. The nurse is reinforc-
    ing teaching related to a low-fat diet. Which
    of the following foods are included in a
    low-fat diet?
    a. cheese omelet
    b. egg salad sandwich
    c. peanut butter
    d. roast beef

62. A client with a delusional disorder believes he is missing all the fingers from his right hand. The nurse assists in planning care for this client with which subtype of delusional disorder?
   a. conjugal
   b. erotomania
   c. persecutory
   d. somatic

63. The nurse is caring for a female client diagnosed with Cushing's disease. The client needs to modify her dietary intake to control symptoms. In addition to restricting sodium, which of the following strategies is most appropriate?
   a. increasing caloric intake
   b. increasing protein intake
   c. restricting fat intake by 10%
   d. restricting potassium intake

64. The nurse is assessing a client with chronic pain. Which of the following are expected physical assessment findings? Select all that apply.

   1. depression
   2. elevated vital signs
   3. grimacing
   4. physical inactivity
   5. normal facial expressions
   6. normal vital signs

65. The nurse is participating in the care of a male client diagnosed with gout. Due to the client's diagnosis, the nurse knows that he should avoid which of the following foods? Select all that apply.
   1. chocolate
   2. milk
   3. mussels
   4. salmon
   5. sardines
   6. turkey
   a. 1, 6
   b. 2, 3, 4
   c. 1, 2, 4, 5
   d. 3, 4, 5, 6

66. The LPN is participating in the care of a male client with schizophrenia who is being prepared for discharge. The client tells the nurse that he is homeless and has no family. Which of the following actions is most appropriate?
   a. ensuring the client is referred to social services
   b. documenting the client's situation
   c. inquiring about how the client feels about his living situation
   d. providing the client with names and numbers for local shelters

67. The nurse is working in the postpartum unit. To facilitate maternal infant bonding, the nurse encourages the mother to
   a. attend to the baby each time it cries.
   b. breast-feed the baby in the mother's bed.
   c. keep the baby in the nursery.
   d. use a high-pitched voice to soothe the infant.

68. The nurse is participating in the care of a client who has just completed an alcohol rehabilitation program. Which of the following statements if made by the client indicates an understanding of discharge care?
   a. "I am really going to try to not drink."
   b. "I can have a couple of beers, but no vodka."
   c. "I can't wait to see all my old friends and hang out."
   d. "I found two different places that have AA meetings."

69. An elderly client in an acute care facility is prescribed the benzodiazepine (Ativan). Because of the potential adverse reactions to the medication, the nurse should
   a. assist the client with ambulating.
   b. encourage coughing and deep breathing.
   c. encourage the use of adult diapers.
   d. put the client in a vest restraint.

70. The LPN is caring for a female client who has recently lost her vision. The nurse recognizes that which of the following is the best type of recreational activity for the client?
   a. listening to television
   b. listening to music or a radio show
   c. talking with other clients on the unit
   d. reading material that is set in Braille

71. A parent brings her 13-year-old son to a clinic and states that she is worried because the boy has not yet started puberty and her friend's daughter started puberty when she was 11. The nurse's best response is which of the following?
   a. "He needs additional testing."
   b. "I will bring your concern to the doctor."
   c. "My son started puberty at 12."
   d. "Onset of puberty in boys is at 13 to 15."

72. The LPN is caring for a child with cerebral palsy. While observing the child eating lunch, the nurse notices the child is having difficulty manipulating the fork and requires assistance. Which of the following is the most appropriate referral for the child?
   a. a registered dietitian
   b. an occupational therapist
   c. social services
   d. a registered nurse

73. The licensed practical nurse is working in the labor and delivery unit when he notices a fetal heart rate showing the following in the fetal monitor.

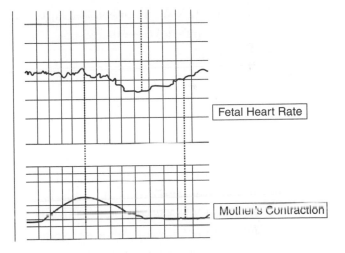

The nurse notifies the registered nurse that the monitor is showing
   a. early decelerations.
   b. late decelerations.
   c. normal fetal patterns.
   d. variable decelerations.

74. The LPN is observing a nursing assistant caring for an 11-month-old infant. Which of the following is incorrect if observed by the LPN?
    a. Before the infant's bath the room temperature is set at 75 degrees F.
    b. The infant's bathwater temperature is checked with the nurse's elbow prior to bathing the infant.
    c. The infant's teeth are swabbed with wet gauze.
    d. The infant is dusted with baby powder after the infant is bathed.

75. The nurse working in a postpartum unit is reviewing the chart of a neonate. The chart documents that the neonate's Apgar score was 8 at 1 minute and 9 at 5 minutes. The nurse knows that at birth the neonate required which of the following?
    a. gentle stimulation
    b. no interventions
    c. oxygen
    d. resuscitation

76. The nurse is caring for a client who is receiving digoxin (Lanoxin) and hydrochlorothiazide (HydroDIURIL) for the treatment of heart failure. Which of the following laboratory values is most important for the nurse to monitor because of the client's medication regimen?
    a. complete blood count
    b. cardiac enzymes
    c. serum BUN and creatinine
    d. serum electrolytes

77. The LPN is supervising a nursing assistant during the care of a client diagnosed with acquired immunodeficiency syndrome (AIDS). The assistant voices concerns about her personal safety. What information is most appropriate for the LPN to share with the assistant to ease her concerns?
    a. If the assistant becomes infected, insurance will help pay for needed medications.
    b. The client with AIDS has a longer life expectancy than in the past.
    c. The AIDS virus is spread by bodily fluids and blood.
    d. Wearing gloves can prevent the spread of the HIV virus.

78. The LPN has instructed a nursing assistant (NA) to place a burned child in the prone position. If the NA does as instructed, the LPN will observe the child positioned in which manner?
    a. in a sitting position
    b. on the abdomen
    c. on the back
    d. on the side

79. The nurse is caring for a client who is ordered a lumbar puncture to rule out meningitis. The nurse is helping the physician position the client for the procedure. Which of the following indicates the nurse has placed the client in the correct position?
    a. The client is in the prone position with the head turned to the side.
    b. The client is in the recumbent position with the feet elevated.
    c. The client is in the side-lying position with the knees drawn to the chest.
    d. The client is in the supine position with the head of bed elevated.

80. The nurse is observing an LPN providing care for a male client diagnosed with leukemia. Which of the LPN's actions indicates the need for additional teaching when caring for this client?

   a. maintaining protective isolation precautions

   b. taking the client's temperature orally

   c. using a cotton-tipped swab to clean the client's teeth

   d. utilizing a standard razor and warm towel when shaving the client

81. The nurse is assisting in the assessment of a neonate's reflexes. The nurse documents this response of the infant as the _____ reflex.

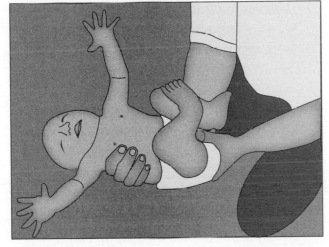

82. The nurse is caring for a client with Cushing's syndrome. The client is ordered a low-sodium diet. How will the nurse monitor for a therapeutic response to the low-sodium diet?

   a. assessing skin turgor

   b. measuring for pedal edema

   c. monitoring sodium intake

   d. weighing the client daily

83. The nurse is participating in the care of a client who is to receive a colostomy. The client is very anxious and nervous about the follow-up care that will be required. Which of the following healthcare providers should be consulted in the care of this client?

   a. the clinical nurse educator

   b. the registered nurse

   c. the social worker

   d. the wound, ostomy, continence nurse

84. The nurse is assisting in childbirth classes. The nurse identifies that risk factors for pre-term delivery include which of the following?

   a. cervical competence

   b. high socioeconomic status

   c. implantation of the embryo

   d. placenta previa

85. The nurse is assisting in the discharge instructions for a client prescribed isocarboxazid (Marplan). The nurse determines that additional teaching is needed when the client states that he should avoid which of the following?

   a. apples

   b. bananas

   c. caffeine

   d. yogurt

86. The nurse has just completed a hospital in-service program on informed consent (IC). Which statement if made by the nurse shows an accurate understanding of IC policy?

   a. "Mentally incompetent clients are permitted to give informed consent."

   b. "It is acceptable for the nurse and/or the physician to obtain informed consent from the client."

   c. "Minors are able to give informed consent if they came to the hospital alone."

   d. "To give informed consent, the client must receive an explanation of the procedure, risks, and benefits."

87. The nurse is participating in the care of a client who is being cared for in an extended care facility. The client is mechanically ventilated and has repeatedly attempted to remove the endotracheal tube. Which of the following restraint devices would be most appropriate for the nursing staff to apply?

a. belt

b. four-point

c. vest

d. wrist

88. A newly hired LPN prepares to administer vitamin K (AquaMEPHYTON) to a newborn. The nurse draws up 1 mg of vitamin K and prepares to administer a subcutaneous injection in the right, lateral anterior thigh. Which of the following actions by the LPN preceptor is indicated in this situation?

a. asking the nurse to stop and reevaluate her injection method

b. keeping the newborn distracted during the injection

c. no actions are required by the LPN preceptor at this time

d. stopping the nurse and having her use the Z-track method for injection

89. A pediatric client is admitted to the nursing unit with a diagnosis of severe gastroenteritis. To prevent the spread of infection, the nurse will

a. ensure standard precautions are implemented.

b. place the child in a semiprivate room.

c. sterilize the client's eating utensils after meals.

d. single-bag all the child's linens.

90. The nurse is participating in the care of a 7-month-old male child being prepared for discharge following a urinary stent procedure to repair a hypospadias. The nurse will reinforce which of the following teaching points to the child's parents?

a. Clean the tip of the penis 3 times daily with soap and water.

b. Measure the child's urinary output from the drainage bag.

c. Avoid giving the child fruit juices.

d. Do not bathe the child until the stent is removed.

91. The nurse is participating in the care of an elderly nursing home client with escalating dementia. The client was been wandering the nursing unit at night and has an unsteady gait. As a result, the client has fallen three times with no resultant injuries. The most appropriate action for the nurse to take is which of the following?

a. Help the client to and from bed and ensure all four side bedrails are raised.

b. Inquire whether the client's family members can stay with the client at night.

c. Place the client in a room closer to the nurse's station and apply a bed alarm.

d. Place the client in a reclining chair across from the nurse's station at night.

92. The licensed practical nurse (LPN) is assisting a registered nurse who is conducting a childbirth class. The LPN determines that the participants have understood the content when the participants indicate which of the following is a sign of false labor?

a. bloody show

b. intensity increases with ambulation

c. irregular contractions

d. progressive dilation of the cervix

93. The nurse is assisting in the planning of care for a client who stopped his selective serotonin reuptake inhibitor (SSRI) because he felt he no longer needed it. The nurse includes monitoring for the side effects relating to suddenly stopping the medication. These include all EXCEPT which of the following?
    a. constipation
    b. diarrhea
    c. euphoria
    d. headaches

94. The nurse is assisting in the development of an injury prevention program for adolescents. The nurse knows that the number-one cause of accidental injuries in high school students is
    a. alcohol consumption.
    b. domestic violence.
    c. motor vehicle accidents.
    d. substance abuse.

95. The nurse is working in a nursing home. The facility has instituted a falls prevention program. Which of the following nursing actions will most likely assure the highest level of fall prevention?
    a. ensuring "Fall Risk" signs are posted outside the clients' rooms
    b. having clients wear colored armbands that indicate that a fall risk
    c. making frequent rounds of the unit and clients' rooms
    d. positioning the clients' beds in the lowest position

96. A client tells a nurse working in the postpartum unit that she is afraid to breast-feed her infant because her sister contracted a very painful mastitis when she was breast-feeding. The nurse knows that which of the following strategies can help to prevent mastitis?
    a. completely emptying the breast at each feeding
    b. consistently feeding the infant on same breast
    c. utilization of improper latching-on technique
    d. use of a hand sanitizer versus soap and water

97. The nurse has just been trained on how to use and care for a blood glucose monitor (glucometer). Which of the following nursing interventions demonstrates proper use of a blood glucose monitor?
    a. The nurse recalibrates the monitor after new batteries are inserted.
    b. The nurse removes her gloves after removing the test strip from the monitor.
    c. The nurse smears the blood sample on the test strip.
    d. The nurse obtains the blood sample directly after cleansing the digit with alcohol.

98. The nurse is completing a home care visit for a client with hepatitis A. The nurse recognizes that the client understands how to prevent transmission if the client focuses on which of the following?
    a. alpha-interferon
    b. condom usage
    c. insulin syringe disposal
    d. proper food handling

99. Which of the following images is an example of medical asepsis? Select all that apply.

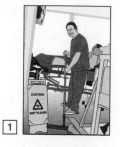
1

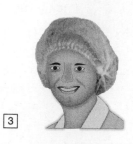
3

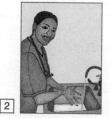
2

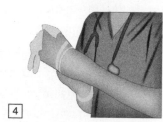
4

    a. 1, 2, 3, 4
    b. 2, 3, 4
    c. 1, 2
    d. 3

100. The licensed practical nurse and a registered nurse are conducting a program for high school students on sexually transmitted infections (STIs). After the program has concluded, a 15-year-old girl tells the nurse that she is pregnant and that she has not received prenatal care. The girl admits to smoking and drinking but denies illicit drug use. The nurse's priority is to help the girl

    a. find prenatal care.
    b. quit drinking.
    c. quit smoking.
    d. tell her parents.

101. The nurse is ordered to administer an intramuscular injection of Rhogam to a woman in preterm labor. The following picture shows the nurse palpating the client's abdomen. At which site indicated on the image should the nurse administer the injection?

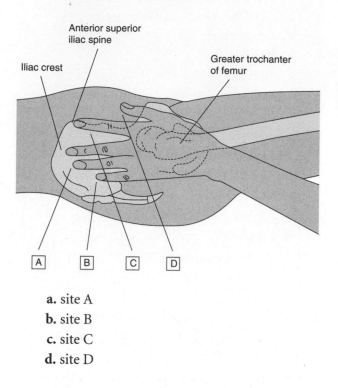

    a. site A
    b. site B
    c. site C
    d. site D

102. A woman is three days post ostomy surgery. The client will not make eye contact with the nurse and does not want any visitors. The nurse recognizes which of the following coping mechanisms?

    a. anxiety
    b. depression
    c. distancing
    d. refusing care

103. The nurse working in a pediatric clinic is helping the registered nurse conduct a developmental assessment on a 5-month-old. The nurse determines that the infant may need additional evaluation upon noting that the infant demonstrates which of the following behaviors?
a. cannot build a 4-block tower
b. grasps objects voluntarily
c. strong palmar grasp reflex
d. well-developed pincer grasp

104. The nurse is caring for a client on an orthopedic unit. While the nurse is ambulating with the client in the hallway, the client falls. Which of the following is the nurse's first responsibility in this situation?
a. assess the client for injuries
b. complete an incident report per hospital policy
c. notify the client's healthcare provider
d. notify the nurse manager of the fall

105. The nurse is administering Rhogam to a pregnant woman. The nurse knows that the medication has been effective when
a. the fetus produces Rh antibodies.
b. the fetus produces no Rh antibiodies.
c. the mother produces Rh antibodies.
d. the mother produces no Rh antibodies.

106. The nurse recognizes that when he or she commits an act of negligence while caring for a client, it is termed
a. criminal negligence.
b. malpractice.
c. misdemeanor.
d. tort.

107. The nurse has just received the client report for her nursing shift. Which of the clients should the nurse see first?
a. a client requiring a dressing change
b. a client requiring oral suctioning
c. a client who is incontinent and needs cleansing
d. a client who needs medication for incisional pain

108. A licensed practical nurse is helping the registered nurse plan an educational program on Dr. Elisabeth Kubler-Ross's stages of grief. The nurse plans the program knowing that the order in which the stages occur is denial, anger, _____, depression, acceptance.

109. The nurse is preparing to administer prostaglandin E to a pregnant woman who is in the early stages of labor. When the client asks the nurse the purpose of the medication, the nurse responds that prostaglandin E helps to
a. ease pain from contractions.
b. prevent cervical infection.
c. ripen the cervix for delivery.
d. prevent postpartum bleeding.

110. The nurse must give a client a tepid sponge bath to lower the client's temperature/fever. Which of the following temperature readings is most appropriate for tepid water?
a. 110 degrees F
b. 105 degrees F
c. 90 degrees F
d. 65 degrees F

111. The nurse is working in a physician's office. A client presents complaining of gallbladder pain. On the image shown here, identify the gallbladder.

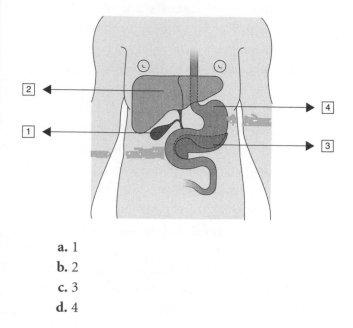

a. 1
b. 2
c. 3
d. 4

112. The licensed practical nurse is working on a postpartum unit and the registered nurse asks her to be sure that the antidote for magnesium sulfate toxicity is readily available for a client receiving it. The licensed practical nurse looks for which medication?

a. calcium gluconate
b. Methergine
c. Narcan
d. Rhogam

113. The nurse is administering an intramuscular injection to a toddler. Which site should the nurse avoid using?

a. deltoid
b. dorsal gluteal
c. rectus femoris
d. vastis lateralis

114. The nurse is assisting in the planning of care for a client with antisocial personality disorder. The nurse includes assessment for which of the following in the plan of care?

a. changes in appetite
b. low energy levels
c. manipulative behavior
d. repetitive hand motions

115. The nurse is completing an assessment on a neonate and notices that the infant's head shows a swelling of the soft tissues between the bone and periosteum. The swelling does not cross the suture lines. The nurse documents the presence of which of the following?

a. anencephaly
b. caput succedaneum
c. cephalohematoma
d. Dandy-Walker syndrome

116. The nurse is assessing pedal pulses on her assigned client. On the image shown here, the nurse is assessing which of the following?

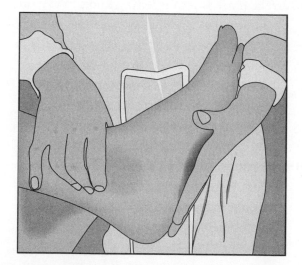

a. dorsalis pedis pulse
b. femoral pulse
c. popliteal pulse
d. posterior tibial pulse

117. The licensed practical nurse is assisting the registered nurse in a community health program about anorexia and bulimia. The nurse realizes that additional teaching is needed when a participant states that the risk factors for anorexia include which of the following?
   a. low self-esteem
   b. model-child syndrome
   c. Russel's sign
   d. sexual abuse

118. The nurse is caring for a child with an arm board in place to secure IV access. The arm board is taped in position. To provide care for the child, the nurse should do which of the following?
   a. leave the arm board in place while providing care
   b. remove the arm board and clean the child's arm
   c. remove one piece of tape at time while bathing the child's arm
   d. remove the arm board and perform range of motion exercises

119. The nurse is participating in the care of a client who experienced a pulmonary embolus, which has resolved. Which of the following instructions should the nurse give the client?
   a. "Always sit with your legs lower than the rest of your body."
   b. "It is important to limit your fluid to one liter a day."
   c. "Tell the staff if your legs swell, or are painful, red, and/or warm."
   d. "Walking is very important; walk at least every other day."

120. The nurse is participating in the care of a client who is diagnosed with breast cancer. The client is also diagnosed with an anxiety disorder. The nurse understands that which of the following client goals will provide the best long-term outcome?
   a. The client will aim to keep follow-up appointments with psychiatrists.
   b. The client will aim to solve problems without help from others.
   c. The client will aim to take medications as prescribed.
   d. The client will aim to understand the side effects of medications.

121. The nurse is assisting in a class on pregnancy and fetal development. The nurse demonstrates that at 20 weeks gestation, the fundus will be located at which point in the image?

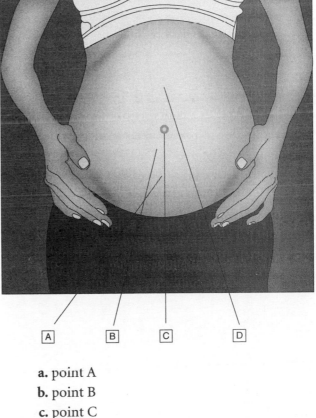

   a. point A
   b. point B
   c. point C
   d. point D

122. The nurse is administering medications on a telemetry unit. A client is ordered 5 mg of oral sustained-release nitroglycerin (Nitro-Time). The medication is supplied in 2.5 mg tablets. How many tablets will the nurse administer?

a. 2

b. 2.5

c. 3

d. 4

123. The licensed practical nurse (LPN) measuring the head and chest circumference of a neonate obtains a head circumference of 36 cm and chest circumference of 31 cm. The LPN reports the measurements to the registered nurse because this may be indicative of

a. caput succedaneum.

b. cephalohematoma.

c. hydrocephalus.

d. molding.

124. The nurse is caring for a mental health client who is extremely angry. The nurse recognizes which of the following physiologic responses is unlikely to occur when the client is angry?

a. decreased blood pressure

b. decreased peristalsis

c. increased muscle tension

d. increased respiratory rate

125. The nurse is taking the apical heart rate of a toddler (26-months-old). On the image shown here, identify where the nurse will assess the apical pulse.

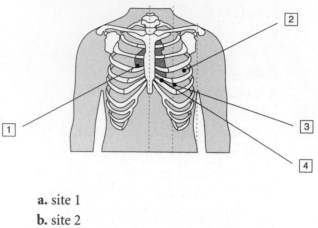

a. site 1

b. site 2

c. site 3

d. site 4

126. The nurse is participating in the care of a client admitted to the detoxification unit for alcohol withdrawal. Which of the following should the nurse do to help the client become sober?

a. have the client drink black coffee

b. have the client take cold showers throughout the day

c. provide the client with a quiet environment for sleeping

d. walk the client around the nursing unit often

127. The parent of a preschooler comes to the physician's office due to the child's having flu-like symptoms. The mother asks the nurse why the doctor said not to give the child aspirin. The nurse responds that when children with flu-like symptoms or chickenpox are given aspirin, they have an increased risk for

a. appendicitis.

b. an asthma attack.

c. Reye's syndrome.

d. rheumatic fever.

128. The nurse is working with a client who is diagnosed with depression. The client tells the nurse that he is thinking of killing himself. The nurse should

    a. ask whether he has a plan.

    b. ask whether he has a will.

    c. avoid talking about it.

    d. tell him he has a lot to live for.

129. The nurse is participating in the care of an infant who has just undergone the surgical correction of pyloric stenosis. While the infant's mother is standing at the infant's crib she says, "If I just would have brought my baby to the hospital sooner, maybe the surgery could have been avoided." Which of the following is the nurse's best response?

    a. "Do you feel that your baby's health problems indicate that you are not a good mother?"

    b. "Do you think that earlier hospitalization could have avoided surgery?"

    c. "Please try not to worry, your baby is going to be just fine."

    d. "Surgery is the most effective treatment for pyloric stenosis."

130. The nurse is participating in the care of a female client who had mitral valve surgery four days ago. The client states, "I keep hearing a clicking nose in my chest and my incision is very large." The nurse recognizes the client may be experiencing which of the following?

    a. altered tissue perfusion

    b. anxiety related to altered body image

    c. anxiety related to hospitalization

    d. knowledge deficit related to postoperative course

131. The nurse is caring for a client who had a recent below-the-knee amputation of the right leg. The client tells the nurse, "I hate the idea of now being a cripple." Which of the following is the most therapeutic response by the nurse?

    a. "Once the physician provides you with more postoperative teaching, you'll feel better."

    b. "Tell me more about how you are feeling."

    c. "You are very lucky to have a large family to take care of you."

    d. "You still have one functional leg."

132. The nurse is participating in the care of a client diagnosed with Addison's disease. The client's condition has stabilized. The client asks the nurse, "I have a very stressful job; how can I manage all my stress?" The nurse's response should include which of the following recommendations?

    a. avoid talking about stressful experiences or situations

    b. remove all stressors from daily living

    c. take antianxiety medications daily as ordered

    d. utilize relaxation techniques such as music

133. The nurse is caring for a client who had a total hip replacement five days ago. The client states concerns about the possibility of dislocating the prosthesis. The nurse should respond to the client by stating which of the following?

    a. "Decreasing the use of the abductor pillow will strengthen the hip muscles and help prevent dislocation."

    b. "You have nothing to worry about; your new hip is very sturdy."

    c. "You should avoid activities that cause adduction to the hip."

    d. "Using a toilet set that is cushioned will help prevent a dislocation."

134. The nurse is assisting in a hearing screening. The LPN is directed by the registered nurse to perform the Weber test. The LPN should implement the test by

   a. standing 18 inches behind client and whispering a statement.

   b. standing 18 inches in front of the client and whispering a statement.

   c. striking a tuning fork and placing it midline on the parietal bone.

   d. striking a tuning fork and placing it on the mastoid process.

135. The nurse is assisting in the care of a 10-week-old infant with pyloric stenosis. The nurse expects the child to exhibit

   a. absent rooting reflex.

   b. decreased suck reflex.

   c. spitting up after feedings.

   d. vomiting after feedings.

136. A nurse is caring for a client who has just returned to the medical-surgical unit from the recovery room after a left hip arthroplasty. The nurse's first intervention should be to check the client's

   a. airway patency.

   b. blood pressure.

   c. heart rate.

   d. left hip dressing.

137. The nurse is reviewing a client's lab values and determines that which result is abnormal?

   a. blood urea nitrogen (BUN) 22 mg/dL

   b. fasting glucose 100 mg/dL

   c. sodium 130 mEq/L

   d. potassium 5 mEq/L

138. The nurse is caring for a client who is prescribed Azelex (azelaic acid). The nurse recognizes this medication is used to treat which of the following?

   a. acne

   b. eczema

   c. excessive hair growth

   d. herpes simplex

139. The nurse is completing an assessment on a client. The nurse is auscultating the client's breath sounds. On the image shown here, identify the area where the nurse should auscultate bronchovesicular breath sounds.

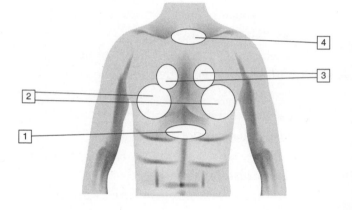

   a. site 1

   b. site 2

   c. site 3

   d. site 4

140. A nurse is entering a client's room and finds the client on the floor of the room. The nurse's priority action is to

   a. assess consciousness.

   b. assist the client back to bed.

   c. call the client's family.

   d. call the client's physician.

141. A child with tetralogy of Fallot begins to cry and becomes cyanotic while the nurse is in the room. The nurse should place the child in which position?
   a. knee-chest
   b. right lateral
   c. standing
   d. Trendelenburg

142. A client is in contact precautions due to a C. diff infection. The nurse should include which of the following in her or his plan of care when taking the client's vital signs. Select all that apply.
   1. gloves
   2. gown
   3. hand sanitizer
   4. mask
   a. 1, 2
   b. 1, 3
   c. 1, 4
   d. 2, 4

143. A client asks the nurse about food choices on the Dietary Approaches to Stop Hypertension (DASH) diet. The nurse responds that which of the following foods should be limited/avoided?
   a. canned vegetables
   b. frozen fruits
   c. lean meats
   d. low-fat yogurts

144. The nurse is administering donepezil (Aricept) to a client. The nurse knows that this medication is used for clients with
   a. alcohol abuse.
   b. Alzheimer's disease.
   c. depression.
   d. psychotic symptoms.

145. The nurse is working with a client with hypertension who is ordered digoxin (Lanoxin) 0.25 mg daily. The client's heart rate is 45 beats per minute. The nurse should
   a. administer the digoxin and document the pulse.
   b. administer the digoxin and call the doctor.
   c. administer the digoxin and call a code.
   d. hold the digoxin and notify the doctor.

146. The nurse is measuring an infant's head circumference. Where should the nurse place the tape measure?
   a. across the eyebrows
   b. at the hairline
   c. at the center of the forehead
   d. over the eyes

147. The nurse is administering a client's 9 a.m. medications. The nurse stops and contacts the physician when he or she notices that the client is ordered which of the following?
   a. metformin (Glucophage) and phenelzine sulfate (Nardil)
   b. metformin (Glucophage) and sertraline (Zoloft)
   c. phenelzine sulfate (Nardil) and sertraline (Zoloft)
   d. phenelzine sulfate (Nardil) and cetirizine (Zyrtek)

148. A nurse is discussing living wills and advance directives with a client when the client asks how often a living will should be updated. The nurse answers that the living will should be reviewed every
   a. month.
   b. year.
   c. 5 years.
   d. 10 years.

149. The nurse is caring for a client with a diabetic foot ulcer in the acute care setting. The nurse would expect which of the following to be involved in the client's care?

   a. nutritionist

   b. occupational therapist

   c. recreational therapist

   d. risk manager

150. The nurse is assisting in a staff development program on antipsychotic medications. It is determined that additional teaching is needed when a participant states that symptoms of drug-induced Parkinson's disease include

   a. flat affect.

   b. shuffling gait.

   c. toe tapping.

   d. tremors.

151. The nurse is reading the chart of an 8-month-old infant and notices that the child is documented to have a café au lait spot. The nurse expects to find

   a. bluish-black spots on the buttocks and sacrum.

   b. a dark-red spot with irregular borders.

   c. an oval or round light-brown birthmark.

   d. tiny white sebaceous glands across the nose.

152. A pregnant client asks the nurse: "What is this dark line running down my abdomen?" The nurse responds appropriately with which of the following?

   a. linea nigra

   b. melasma

   c. Montgomery tubercles

   d. striae gravidarum

153. A client comes to the emergency room after attempting suicide. The nurse should

   a. administer a sedative for sleep.

   b. ensure one-to-one observation.

   c. place the client in isolation precautions.

   d. place the client in a vest restraint.

154. A nurse works on a medical-surgical floor of an acute care facility. The emergency room has become extremely busy and the nurse is told to report to the emergency room for the remainder of her shift. The nurse has not been oriented to the emergency room (ER). The nurse should report to the ER and

   a. refuse the assignment.

   b. contact the hospital's vice president of nursing.

   c. identify what tasks she or he can safely perform and consult with the ER charge nurse/manager.

   d. perform only the duties of a nursing aide.

155. The nurse is assessing an infant for changes in intracranial pressure (ICP). The nurse recognizes it is important to palpate the infant's fontanels. On the image below, identify where the nurse should palpate to make an assessment of the anterior fontanel.

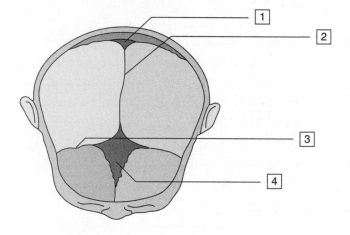

   a. site 1

   b. site 2

   c. site 3

   d. site 4

156. The nurse is contributing to a staff development program on peripheral vascular/arteriole disease. The nurse realizes that additional teaching is needed when a staff member states that it is safe to utilize tightly applied ace wraps on clients exhibiting signs and symptoms of
_____.

157. The nurse is assisting in the discharge teaching of the mother whose child was seen in the emergency room for pinkeye. The nurse determines additional teaching is needed when the mother indicates that she will
a. administer eyedrops as ordered.
b. send the child to school the next day.
c. use cold compresses on the child's eyes.
d. use a separate towel for the infected child.

158. The nurse is reinforcing teaching from the nutritionist regarding appropriate dietary considerations for a client with gastroesophageal reflux disease (GERD). The nurse knows that the client needs additional teaching when the client states he should
a. avoid spicy foods.
b. decrease caffeine intake.
c. eat three meals per day
d. sleep with the upper body elevated.

159. A nursing aide is caring for a client with osteoarthritis and asks the nurse what is wrong with the client's fingers when she notices that the joints just in from the tips of the fingers are hard and knobby. The nurse correctly responds that these are which of the following?

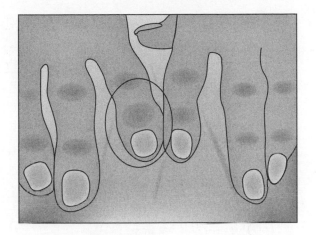

a. Bouchard's nodes
b. Heberden's nodes
c. Hemangioma
d. Mongolian spots

160. The nurse is reinforcing dietary guidelines provided by the nutritionist to a mother whose child was diagnosed with phenylketonuria. The nurse includes that the child should avoid which of the following?
a. aspartame
b. broccoli
c. bananas
d. fructose

161. The nurse is preparing to administer an IM flu shot. Where should the nurse administer the injection?

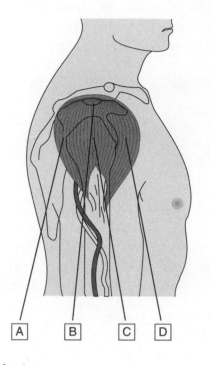

    a. site A
    b. site B
    c. site C
    d. site D

162. The nurse is assisting in providing education to a group of nursing assistants when one of the assistants asks which portion of the brain impacts balance. The nurse correctly answers _____.

163. The nurse is assisting a registered nurse to plan a cancer prevention education program in the community. The nurse includes which of the following as a higher risk factor for breast cancer?
    a. first period at age 13
    b. not breast-feeding children
    c. having more than 5 children
    d. exercising frequently and not being overweight

164. The physician orders collagenase (Santyl) to be placed on a client's stage-3 pressure ulcer on the sacrum. Where is the client's sacrum located?

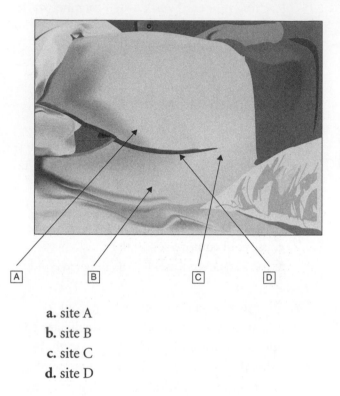

    a. site A
    b. site B
    c. site C
    d. site D

165. The nurse is assisting in a staff workshop on the prevention of nosocomial infections. The nurse determines that the participants understand the concepts when they state the best intervention for the prevention of nosocomial infections is which of the following?
    a. use of gowns
    b. use of gloves
    c. hand hygiene
    d. sterile technique

Answers

1. a. CPM is a modality of postoperative treatment intended to assist recovery following joint surgery or injuries of the upper or lower extremities. CPM equipment covers a range of mechanical devices designed to move the client's joint or extremity without the use of the client's muscles through a prescribed range of motion over extended periods of time. Further teaching is indicated if the nurse states that CPM is unnecessary if he is receiving PT, as these therapies are both needed for optimal recovery. Choice **b** is incorrect. CPM as well as PT aid in preventing adhesions. Choice **c** is incorrect. The client's skin should be assessed while the CPM device is in place. Choice **d** is incorrect. Bleeding is a complication associated with the CPM devices, therefore it is appropriate for the nurse to assess for bleeding when the device is in use.

Category: Safe and Effective Care Environment: Coordination of Care

Subcategory: Adult: Musculoskeletal Disorders

2. d. Antianxiety medication doses may be increased during treatment to maintain comfort throughout the dying process. Choice **a** is incorrect. Palliative care focuses on keeping the client comfortable; pain medication will most likely be increased as needed throughout the dying process. Choice **b** is incorrect. Palliative care focuses on keeping the client comfortable; oxygen therapy will most likely stay the same or be increased as needed. Choice **c** is incorrect. Palliative care focuses on keeping the client comfortable. The administration of increased IV fluids and oral fluids is often individualized based on the client's specific circumstances and is not generally an assumed aspect of palliative care.

Category: Safe and Effective Care Environment: Coordination of Care

Subcategory: Adult: Renal Disorders

3. The correct answer is *June 22, 2013*.

To use Naegele's rule, subtract three months from the first day of the last menstrual period and add seven days. One year is added as needed. In this case, the calculation is as follows. September minus three months is June. Fifteen plus seven days is twenty-two. Since the period between September and June includes January, one year is also added making the due date June 22, 2013.

Category: Physiological Integrity: Basic Care and Comfort

Subcategory: Maternal Infant: Antepartum

4. b. Regression occurs when one reverts to an earlier stage of development due to stress. The boy regressed back to bed-wetting due to the stress of the parents' separation. Choice **a** is incorrect. Passive aggression occurs when one expresses aggression indirectly. Choice **c** is incorrect. Repression occurs when a painful thought or memory is involuntarily excluded from one's memory. Choice **d** is incorrect. Suppression occurs when a painful thought or memory is intentionally excluded from one's memory.
Category: Psychosocial Integrity
Subcategory: Mental Health: Defense Mechanisms

5. c. The nurse should remember "clear then cloudy." When preparing a mixture of regular insulin with insulin of another type, such as NPH insulin, the regular (clear) insulin is drawn up in the syringe first. This practice/sequence of actions will avoid contaminating the vial of regular insulin with insulin of another type. Choices **a**, **b**, and **d** are correct practices for preparing NPH and regular insulin in the same syringe.
Category: Physiological Integrity: Pharmacology
Subcategory: Adult Endocrine Disorders

6. d. The ECG tracing is ventricular tachycardia (VT). In VT, the heart rate is not measurable; it indicates a medical emergency and a code should be initiated promptly. Choice **a** is incorrect. This ECG tracing is not atrial fibrillation; it is ventricular tachycardia (VT). Choice **b** is incorrect. This ECG tracing is not atrial flutter; it is ventricular tachycardia (VT). Choice **c** is incorrect. This ECG tracing is not ventricular fibrillation; it is ventricular tachycardia (VT).
Category: Physiological Integrity: Physiological Adaptation
Subcategory: Adult Cardiovascular Disorders

7. c. The fetal heartbeat can be heard with a Doppler at 10 to 12 weeks. Choice **a** is incorrect. This is too early to hear the fetal heartbeat with a Doppler; the fetal heartbeat is commonly heard between 10 and 12 weeks. Choice **b** is incorrect. While the heartbeat may be heard at 9 weeks, it is more commonly heard between 10 and 12 weeks. Choice **d** is incorrect. This is too late. The fetal heartbeat is commonly heard by Doppler between 10 and 12 weeks.
Category: Physiological Integrity: Physiological Adaptation
Subcategory: Maternal Infant: Fetal Development

8. c. Protection from droplet transmission requires the nurse to wear a mask. Choice **a** is incorrect. A gown is required for protection from contact transmission. Choice **b** is incorrect. Gloves are required for protection from contact transmission. Choice **d** is incorrect. A respiratory protective device is needed to protect against airborne transmission.
Category: Safe and Effective Care Environment: Safety and Infection Control
Subcategory: Adult: Respiratory Disorders

9. b. By stating, "I will stay here with you," the nurse is offering the client emotional support. Choice **a** is incorrect. The nurse should allow the client to express her feelings; the nurse cannot assure the client in this situation that everything will be okay. Choice **c** is incorrect. This statement takes the focus off the client and her needs and inappropriately directs the focus to the nurse. Choice **d** is incorrect. This is an inappropriate response. It is not up to the nurse to decide that the client needs a second opinion; rather, the nurse should offer emotional support by offering to stay with the client.
Category: Physiological Integrity: Basic Care and Comfort
Subcategory: Mental Health: Therapeutic Communication

10. b. NPH insulin is an intermediate-acting insulin; therefore, a hypoglycemic reaction will most likely occur during its peak time, which is 4 to 12 hours.
Category: Physiological Integrity: Pharmacology
Subcategory: Adult: Endocrine Disorders

11. d. The focus of therapeutic communication is to facilitate the client's insight into his or her thoughts and feelings. By stating: "You should . . ." the nurse is telling the client what to do versus allowing the client to explore his or her thoughts and feelings. Choice **a** is incorrect. This phrasing aims to clarify what the client is stating and will foster the therapeutic relationship. Choice **b** is incorrect. This phrasing restates what the client has said to ensure that the nurse correctly understands the client's meaning. Restating is a therapeutic communication technique. Choice **c** is incorrect. This is an example of an open-ended statement. This type of statement fosters the therapeutic relationship.
Category: Psychosocial Integrity
Subcategory: Mental Health: Therapeutic Communication

12. c. Zofran is an antiemetic that is used to treat nausea and vomiting. Choice **a** is incorrect. Zofran is not used to treat gastrointestinal irritation; it is an antiemetic that is used to treat nausea and vomiting. Choice **b** is incorrect. Zofran is not used to treat incisional pain; it is an antiemetic that is used to treat nausea and vomiting. Choice **d** is incorrect. Zofran is not used to treat urinary retention; it is an antiemetic that is used to treat nausea and vomiting.
Category: Physiological Integrity: Pharmacology
Subcategory: Adult Gastrointestinal Disorders

13. The correct answer is *autonomy versus shame and doubt.*
An 18-month-old child is a toddler. In Erickson's theory, the stage for toddlerhood is autonomy versus shame and doubt.
Category: Psychosocial Integrity
Subcategory: Pediatrics: Toddlers

14. d. The therapeutic range for a serum digoxin level is 0.5–2.0 ng/mL.
Category: Physiological Integrity: Pharmacology
Subcategory: Adult: Cardiovascular Disorders

15. c. One of the symptoms of burnout is irritability. Choice **a** is incorrect. Empathy is the ability to understand another's feelings and is not a symptom of burnout. Choice **b** is incorrect. A person experiencing burnout will have fatigue, not increased energy. Choice **d** is incorrect. A person experiencing burnout will have a negative outlook versus being optimistic.
Category: Psychosocial Integrity
Subcategory: Mental Health: Stress

16. a. A client experiencing anxiety would have increased urinary frequency, not decreased urinary output. Choice **b** is incorrect. Elevated blood pressure is a symptom of anxiety. Choice **c** is incorrect. Shallow respirations are a symptom of anxiety. Choice **d** is incorrect. Tremors are a symptom of anxiety.
Category: Physiological Adaptation
Subcategory: Mental Health: Anxiety

17. Answer: The nurse would divide 6,000 units by 10,000 units and administer 0.6 mL.
Category: Physiological Integrity: Pharmacology
Subcategory: Adult: Miscellaneous Disorders

18. c. Choice **c** is correct. A client of advanced maternal age (over the age of 35) is at risk for placenta previa. Choice **a** is incorrect. Advanced maternal age (over the age of 35) does not predispose the pregnant woman to anemia. Risk factors include poor nutrition and multiple pregnancies. Choice **b** is incorrect. Risk factors for hyperemesis gravidarum include being overweight and first time pregnancy. Advanced maternal age (over the age of 35) does not predispose the pregnant woman to hyperemesis gravidarum. Choice **d** is incorrect. Risk factors for post-term delivery (delivery after 42 weeks gestation) include prior uterine surgery and prior deliveries but not advanced maternal age (over the age of 35).
Category: Physiological Integrity: Reduction of Risk
Subcategory: Maternal Infant: Maternal Complications

19. c. One teaspoon equals 5 mLs; therefore, the nurse will administer 10 mLs.
Category: Physiological Integrity: Pharmacology
Subcategory: Adult: Gastrointestinal Disorders

20. b. Early ambulation is the most significant general nursing measure to prevent postoperative complications. Walking the client increases vital capacity, maintains normal respiratory functioning, stimulates circulation, prevents venous stasis, improves gastrointestinal and genitourinary function, increases muscle tone, and increases wound healing. Choice **a** is incorrect. Bladder and bowel monitoring is necessary, but early ambulation is the most important intervention. Choice **c** is incorrect. Pain management is necessary, but early ambulation is the most important intervention. Choice **d** is incorrect. A progressive diet is necessary, but early ambulation is the most important intervention.

Category: Physiological Integrity: Reduction of Risk

Subcategory: Adult: Gastrointestinal Disorders

21. Answer: 147.32 cm

One inch equals 2.54 cm. In this equation:

x cm $= \frac{2.54 \text{ cm}}{1 \text{ inch}} \times 58$ inches $=$ $2.54 \times 58 = 147.32$ cm.

Category: Physiological Integrity: Basic Care and Comfort

Subcategory: Pediatric: General Survey

22. c. The nurse recognizes the client may have appendicitis. A CBC should be obtained to determine whether the white blood cell count is elevated. An increased WBC is suggestive of appendicitis. Choice **a** is incorrect. An abdominal X-ray is not likely to be completed. A CT scan of the abdomen will likely be ordered. Choice **b** is incorrect. An enema is contraindicated because the client's diagnosis is not confirmed. An enema, if administered, could rupture the appendix if the client has appendicitis. Choice **d** is incorrect. Deep palpitation of the right abdominal quadrant is contraindicated because the client's diagnosis is not confirmed. Deep palpation, if completed, could rupture the appendix if the client has appendicitis.

Category: Physiological Integrity: Reduction of Risk

Subcategory: Adult: Gastrointestinal Disorders

23. a. Agoraphobia is the fear of crowds or open spaces. Choice **b** is incorrect. A fear of death is thanatophobia. Choice **c** is incorrect. A fear of heights is acrophobia. Choice **d** is incorrect. A fear of water is hydrophobia.

Category: Psychological Integrity

Subcategory: Mental Health: Anxiety Disorders

24. b. The home pregnancy test is based on the presence of human chorionic gonadotropin in the urine. Choice **a** is incorrect. Maternal estrogen and progesterone levels are tested through serum levels and they are not the hormone tested for in home pregnancy tests. Choice **c** is incorrect. Follicle stimulation hormone is assessed through blood testing and is not the hormone tested for in home pregnancy tests. Choice **d** is incorrect. Alpha-fetoprotein testing is a part of the screening test for genetic abnormalities in the fetus such as neural tube defects and Down's syndrome.

Category: Physiological Integrity: Basic Care and Comfort

Subcategory: Maternal Health: Antepartum

25. d. Taking nitroglycerin (a vasodilator) prior to sexual intercourse can often prevent chest pains and enhance/improve a male client's erection. Choice **a** is incorrect. Clients taking nitroglycerin should not take ED medication. ED medications are contraindicated because an unsafe drop in blood pressure can occur. Choice **b** is incorrect. Resting prior to sex is not necessary. Choice **c** is incorrect. It is not necessary to avoid sexual activity for five months following an MI.

Category: Physiological Integrity: Reduction of Risk

Subcategory: Adult: Cardiovascular Disorders

26. b. The client is experiencing neuropathy. Neuropathies are commonly seen in clients diagnosed with pernicious anemia. Choice **a** is incorrect. Trouble seeing/being able to read the newspaper is a common problem for clients is their sixties; farsightedness is not unusual during the aging process. Choice **c** is incorrect. Joint pain is not a complication of pernicious anemia. Choice **d** is incorrect. Headaches are not a complication of pernicious anemia.

Category: Physiological Integrity: Reduction of Risk

Subcategory: Adult: Hematological Disorders

27. The correct answer is 2 capsules.

The nurse must convert 0.2 grams to milligrams. To do this using the metric system, convert larger to smaller; multiply by 1,000 or move the decimal three places to the right. When this conversion is completed, 0.2 grams equals 200 mg. The nurse must then use the following formula to calculate the correct dosage:

Desired dosage ÷ capsule(s) = capsule(s) per dose

200 mg ÷ 100 mg capsule = 2 capsules

Category: Physiological Integrity: Pharmacology

Subcategory: Adult: Neurological Disorders

28. b. The nurse should plan to collect the sputum culture during the early morning hours because the concentration of the organism is usually highest in the morning. Choice **a** is incorrect. The nurse is collecting a single sample, not multiple samples. Choice **c** is incorrect. This is contraindicated because many mouthwashes contain alcohol and would kill the organisms. Choice **d** is incorrect. Instructing the client to increase fluid intake would loosen secretions, but is not a feasible option since this would need to occur during the sleeping hours.
Category: Physiological Integrity: Reduction of Risk
Subcategory: Adult: Respiratory Disorders

29. a. It is necessary to assess the client's reading and writing level because the client will need some way to communicate postoperatively. A common method used is for the client to write on a pad. If the client can't write, another method will need to be used/developed. Choice **b** is incorrect. This is unnecessary because the client can hear. Choice **c** is incorrect. The speech therapist may teach the client esophageal speech after surgery; this is not the nurse's responsibility. Choice **d** is incorrect. It is important for the client to know this, but assessing whether the client can read and write and at what level is the priority.
Category: Physiological Integrity: Reduction of Risk
Subcategory: Adult: Respiratory Disorders

30. b. The nurse should take the client to a quiet area where they can explore the cause of his anger. Choice **a** is incorrect. Avoiding the client until he calms down is not appropriate and does not allow the client to explore the source of his displaced anger. Choice **c** is incorrect. Telling the visitor to come earlier next time does not address the client's anger. Choice **d** is incorrect. While having the client go to his room will remove him from the situation, it will not allow the client to explore and understand the cause of his anger.
Category: Physiological Integrity: Basic Care and Comfort
Subcategory: Mental Health: Therapeutic Communication

31. c. A bronchoscopy is a test to view the airways and diagnose lung disease. It may also be used during the treatment of some lung conditions. The client must be NPO after midnight. Choice **a** is incorrect. There is no need to administer an enema prior to the procedure. Choice **b** is incorrect. The client will be NPO prior to the procedure. Increasing fluids is contraindicated. Choice **d** is incorrect. The client is permitted to take her medications with a sip of water.
Category: Physiological Integrity: Reduction of Risk
Subcategory: Adult: Respiratory Disorders

32. The correct answer is 2,600 − 1,700 = 900 mL. The nurse should subtract the amount of irrigation solution infused into the bladder from the total amount of fluid in the drainage bag.
Category: Physiological Integrity: Reduction of Risk
Subcategory: Adult: Genitourinary Disorders

33. d. Amniocentesis is used to detect neural tube defects. Choice **a** is incorrect. The definitive test for cystic fibrosis is the sweat test (testing for the amount of sodium in the sweat). Choice **b** is incorrect. Amniocentesis does not detect fetal alcohol syndrome. Healthcare providers screen for the risk of fetal alcohol syndrome through assessment of the pregnant woman's alcohol consumption pattern. Choice **c** is incorrect. Meconium aspiration occurs when meconium stool is released into the amniotic fluid and enters into the fetal lungs. This is not detected by amniocentesis, but the fetus is considered at risk for it if there is meconium in the amniotic fluid at the time of delivery.

Category: Health Promotion

Subcategory: Maternal Infant: Antepartum

34. The correct answer is *2, 3, 4, 6.*

The signs and symptoms of hypocalcemia include (depending on the level): seizures; dementia; anxiety; depression; extrapyramidal symptoms (parkinsonism is most common); calcifications of basal ganglia (in longstanding disease); papilledema; increased neuromuscular irritability; Chvostek's sign; Trousseau's sign; paresthesias in the fingers and toes; muscle stiffness, myalgias, and spasms; prolongation of QT interval; congestive heart failure; hypotension; biliary colic; bronchospasms; numbness; dry coarse skin, dermatitis, hyperpigmentation, and eczema; steatorrhea; and gastric achlorhydria. Aphasia is not a sign of hypocalcemia and polyuria is a sign of diabetes mellitus.

Category: Physiological Integrity: Reduction of Risk

Subcategory: Adult: Immune Disorders

35. c. The adolescent should receive 6 teaspoons, according to the following formula.

$$x \text{ teaspoons} = \frac{750 \text{ mg}}{1} \times \frac{10 \text{ mL}}{250 \text{ mg}} \times \frac{1 \text{ tsp}}{5 \text{ mL}}$$
$$= \frac{750 \times 10 \times 1}{1 \times 250 \times 5} = \frac{7,500}{1,250} = 6$$

Choice **a** is incorrect. If the nurse administered 2 teaspoons, the adolescent would receive less than the ordered dose. Choice **b** is incorrect. If the nurse administered 4 teaspoons, the adolescent would receive less than the ordered dose. Choice **d** is incorrect. If the nurse administered 8 teaspoons, the child would receive more than the ordered dose.

Category: Physiological Integrity: Pharmacological Therapies

Subcategory: Pediatrics: Medication

36. d. Since the physician has not specified a solution for irrigation, the nurse should utilize sterile normal saline (NS). The standard of care is sterile NS. Sterile NS is used because the urinary tract is sterile and this isotonic solution will not damage cells. Choice **a** is incorrect. Unsterile solutions should not be used to irrigate the urinary catheter. Choice **b** is incorrect. Hydrogen peroxide is not used to irrigate urinary catheters. Choice **c** is incorrect. Unsterile solutions should not be used to irrigate the urinary catheter.

Category: Physiological Integrity: Physiological Adaptation

Subcategory: Adult: Genitourinary Disorders

37. a. Obstructive jaundice is a condition in which there is a blockage of the flow of bile out of the liver. This results in an overflow of bile and its by-products into the blood, and bile excretion from the body is incomplete. Bilirubin, a component of bile, is yellow, which gives the characteristic yellow appearance of jaundice in the skin, eyes, and mucous membranes. A client diagnosed with obstructive jaundice will experience dark brown urine. Other symptoms of obstructive jaundice include: yellowing of the skin and whites of the eyes; paler/clay colored stools; and intense itching. Choice **b** is incorrect. The stool would be pale and clay colored. Choice **c** is incorrect. Red, dry skin is not associated with obstructive jaundice. Choice **d** is incorrect. Tan, thick sputum is not associated with obstructive jaundice.

Category: Physiological Integrity: Physiological Adaptation

Subcategory: Adult: Hepatic Disorders

38. a. The frontal lobe controls language expression, which is affected by aphasia. Judgment, personality, social behavior, movement, and abstract reasoning are also controlled by the frontal lobe. Choice **b** is incorrect. This is the parietal lobe, which helps in a client's sense of space and ability to navigate; it does not control speech. Choice **c** is incorrect. This is the temporal lobe, which is involved in a range of functions, including emotion and sensory input; it does not control speech. Choice **d** is incorrect. This is the occipital lobe, which affects vision; it does not control speech.

Category: Physiological Integrity: Physiological Adaptation

Subcategory: Adult: Neurological Disorders

39. b. Lochia rubra is the normal occurrence of bloody discharge for the first three days in the postpartum period. Choice **a** is incorrect. If the client was hemorrhaging, she would have uncontrolled vaginal bleeding not simply bloody discharge, a normal occurrence in the early postpartum period. Choice **c** is incorrect. If the client were experiencing subinvolution of the uterus, profuse or prolonged vaginal bleeding would occur. Choice **d** is incorrect. If the client were experiencing uterine infection, other signs of infection such as a foul-smelling lochia, yellow- or green-tinged lochia, and/or fever would be present. Bloody discharge is a normal occurrence in the first three days of the postpartum period.

Category: Safe and Effective Care Environment: Coordinated Care

Subcategory: Maternal Infant: Postpartum

40. c. Narcan (naloxone) is the antidote for opioid overdose. Choice **a** is incorrect. Activated charcoal is used to treat some overdoses and poison ingestions but opioid overdoses are treated with Narcan (naloxone). Choice **b** is incorrect. Antabuse (disulfiram) is used to treat chronic alcoholism. Choice **d** is incorrect. Vitamin K is used to treat Coumadin (warfarin) toxicity.

Category: Physiological Integrity: Pharmacology

Subcategory: Mental Health: Substance Abuse

41. a. Intal is an inhaled nonsteroidal antiallergy agent and a mast cell stabilizer. Common side effects include bronchospasms, nasal congestion, cough, wheezing, and throat irritation. Choice **b** is incorrect. This is not a side effect of Intal. Choice **c** is incorrect. Diarrhea is a side effect associated with the oral form of Intal. Other side effects of the oral form include nausea, myalgia, and pruritus. Choice **d** is incorrect. This is not a side effect of Intal.

Category: Physiological Integrity: Pharmacology

Subcategory: Adult: Respiratory Disorders

42. b. The nurse should suspect emphysema. This enlarged chest, referred to as "barrel chest," manifests itself as a constantly overexpanded chest. The disease consists of thinned out lung tissue, with the chest overexpanding in an attempt to better use the remaining lung function. This is a debilitating disease occurring in later age groups. Choice **a** is incorrect. A barrel chest is not a symptom of bronchitis, but of emphysema. Choice **c** is incorrect. A barrel chest is not a symptom of osteomalacia, but of emphysema. Choice **d** is incorrect. A barrel chest is not a symptom of scoliosis, but of emphysema.

Category: Physiological Integrity: Physiological Adaptation

Subcategory: Adult: Respiratory Disorders

43. b. Both rooting and bringing the hand to the mouth are clues of feeding readiness. Choice **a** is incorrect. Rooting is a feeding readiness clue but hiccups are not. Choice **c** is incorrect. Bringing the hand to the mouth is a feeding readiness clue but waving the arms in the air is not. Choice **d** is incorrect. Bringing the hand to the mouth is a feeding readiness clue but hiccups are not.

Category: Physiological Integrity: Basic Care and Comfort

Subcategory: Pediatrics: Infants

44. c. A soft, boggy uterus is most often due to uterine atony. Choice **a** is incorrect. While a soft and boggy uterus can lead to hemorrhaging, there is no indication that this woman is experiencing hemorrhagic shock at this time. Choice **b** is incorrect. Symptoms of retained placenta include fever, foul-smelling discharge, and cramping. Choice **d** is incorrect. Symptoms of uterine inversion include protrusion of the uterus through the vagina.

Category: Safe and Effective Care Environment: Coordinated Care

Subcategory: Maternal Child: Postpartum

45. b. A client who is experiencing a low serum calcium level may experience a prolonged ST or QT interval. Choice **a** is incorrect. A prolonged P wave is not associated with hypocalcemia. Choice **c** is incorrect. A shortened ST segment occurs with a high calcium level. Choice **d** is incorrect. A widened T wave occurs with a high calcium level.

Category: Physiological Integrity: Physiological Adaptation

Subcategory: Adult: Cardiovascular Disorders

46. d. Tinnitus is the most common complaint of clients suffering from an inner ear disorder. Choice **a** is incorrect. Burning in the ear is not associated with inner ear disorders. Choice **b** is incorrect. Hearing loss is not associated with inner ear disorders. Choice **c** is incorrect. Pruritus, or itching, is not associated with inner ear disorders.

Category: Physiological Integrity: Physiological Adaptation

Subcategory: Adult: Ear Disorders

47. d. The client with an ileostomy is at the greatest risk for developing a fluid volume deficit due to increased gastrointestinal tract loss. Choice **a** is incorrect. A client with acute renal failure is at risk of developing fluid volume overload. Choice **b** is incorrect. A client with heart failure is at risk of developing fluid volume overload. Choice **c** is incorrect. A client diagnosed with hypertension is not at risk of developing a fluid volume disorder.
Category: Physiological Integrity: Physiological Adaptation
Subcategory: Adult: Miscellaneous Disorders

48. b. Substance use is the ingestion of a prescription or over-the-counter substance. This client is experiencing substance use as he or she takes the Vicodin as prescribed. Choice **a** is incorrect. If the client was experiencing dependency, he or she would exhibit intermittent or continuous cravings for the Vicodin. Choice **c** is incorrect. Tolerance occurs when the client needs more and more of a substance to achieve the same effect. Choice **d** is incorrect. Withdrawal occurs when the client becomes symptomatic after he or she suddenly stops using a medication/substance.
Category: Physiological Integrity: Basic Care and Comfort
Subcategory: Mental Health: Substance Abuse

49. d. Magical thinking occurs when the child believes that his or her thoughts are all powerful. Choice **a** is incorrect. Animism occurs when the child gives lifelike qualities to inanimate objects. Choice **b** is incorrect. The child demonstrates categorization when she or he can place objects into categories. Choice **c** is incorrect. Conservation is the ability to understand that certain physical characteristics stay the same when outward appearances change. For example, when milk is poured from a tall, skinny glass into a wide, small glass, the child understands that the amount of milk has not changed.
Category: Psychosocial Integrity
Subcategory: Pediatrics: Toddler

50. The correct answer is *cesarean section*. Rupture of the uterus is considered a medical emergency requiring immediate delivery of the fetus by cesarean section.
Category: Safe and Effective Care Environment: Coordinated Care
Subcategory: Maternal Infant: Intrapartum

51. a. Carbon dioxide acts as an acid in the body. Therefore, with an increase in carbon dioxide, there is a corresponding decrease in the pH level.
Category: Physiological Integrity: Physiological Adaptation
Subcategory: Adult: Respiratory Disorders

52. a. The client should initially be offered a clear liquid diet following surgery. This type of diet aids in stimulating peristalsis as well as moistening the mouth and providing fluid and some energy-supplying calories. A clear liquid diet is also the least likely diet to cause nausea and emesis. The client's diet can be progressed based on tolerance. Choice **b** is incorrect. A low-sodium diet is not appropriate in this situation. Choices **c** and **d** are incorrect.
Category: Physiological Integrity: Basic Care and Comfort
Subcategory: Adult: Miscellaneous Disorders

53. c. The most reliable method of determining/confirming the presence of a fecal impaction is a digital examination. The digital examination will confirm hard, dry stool. Choice **a** is incorrect. Assessing for diarrhea is important in relation to fluid and electrolyte imbalances, but it may not be an indication of a fecal impaction. Choice **b** is incorrect. This is an appropriate physical assessment measure, but will not confirm an impaction. Choice **d** is incorrect. This is an appropriate physical assessment measure, but will not confirm an impaction.
Category: Physiological Integrity: Basic Care and Comfort
Subcategory: Adult: Gastrointestinal Disorders

54. c. The chest tube insertion site should quickly be covered to prevent air from entering and reduce the potential for recollapsing the lung. Choice **a** is incorrect. The client's breath sounds should be assessed, but only after a new chest tube is inserted. Choice **b** is incorrect. Having the client hold his breath is a temporary measure; the most appropriate action is to cover the chest tube site. Choice **d** is incorrect. The chest tube becomes unsterile when dislodged and should not be reinserted.
Category: Physiological Integrity: Basic Care and Comfort
Subcategory: Adult: Miscellaneous Disorders

55. a. Feeling competent is not a symptom of postpartum depression; the opposite is often true. Women experiencing postpartum depression are likely to feel incompetence in the face of their new responsibilities as mothers. Choices **b**, **c**, and **d** are incorrect. Feeling hopeless, panic attacks, and sudden outbursts are symptoms of postpartum depression.
Category: Psychosocial
Subcategory: Maternal Infant: Postpartum

56. c. The client's fingernails should be trimmed short to aid in maintaining skin integrity. Patients who experience liver failure have a buildup of bilirubin in their systems that causes severe itching. The bilirubin irritates the sensory nerves of the patient's brain, which interprets this as an itch. Choice **a** is incorrect. Applying cornstarch to the client's skin will aid in absorbing moisture, but will not relieve the client's itching or decrease the risk for skin breakdown. Choice **b** is incorrect. The client is not experiencing an allergic reaction; consequently, the use of hypoallergenic bed sheets is unnecessary. Choice **d** is incorrect. Utilizing warm water can actually increase the client's itching.
Category: Physiological Integrity: Basic Care and Comfort
Subcategory: Adult: Hepatic Disorders

57. b. The common side effects of this medication include: hypotension, or decreased blood pressure, as well as nausea, dizziness, constipation, fatigue, and diarrhea. Choice **a** is incorrect. A decreased blood glucose level is not a side effect this medication. Choice **c** is incorrect. An elevated heart rate is not a side effect of this medication. Choice **d** is incorrect. An elevated temperature is not a side effect of this medication.
Category: Physiological Integrity: Pharmacology
Subcategory: Adult Eye Disorders

58. a. Based on the absence of saliva, pain in the ear area, and prolonged NPO status, the nurse should suspect parotitis. This condition is an inflammation of the parotid gland and often seen with dehydration. The condition can be prevented by providing frequent mouth care, adequate hydration, and/or hard candy. Choice **b** is incorrect. This condition causes bluish-white lesions in the mouth. Choice **c** is incorrect. This condition is inflammation of the mouth and generally produces excessive sputum and mouth pain. Choice **d** is incorrect. This condition causes inflamed gingival tissue and bleeding that may occur by brushing the teeth.
Category: Physiological Integrity: Basic Care and Comfort
Subcategory: Adult Oral Cavity Disorders

59. The correct answer is *fallopian tubes*. The sperm and egg meet in the fallopian tubes where fertilization occurs.
Category: Physiological Integrity: Physiological Adaptation
Subcategory: Maternal Infant: Fetal Development

60. b. The nurse should instruct the client that a reddish-orange discoloration of the urine may occur and can stain clothing. Choice **a** is incorrect. A headache may occur occasionally and does not warrant discontinuation of the medication. Choices **c** and **d** are incorrect. The nurse should relay that the medication should be taken after meals to decrease gastric upset.
Category: Physiological Integrity: Pharmacology
Subcategory: Adult Renal Disorders

61. d. Lean meats such as roast beef, veal, lamb, and well-trimmed pork and ham are low in fat. Fruits are also low in fat. The client who has a cholecystectomy is not required to be on a special diet, but is encouraged to avoid excessive fat intake. Choice **a** is incorrect. Cheese has a high fat content. Choice **b** is incorrect. The dressing used to prepare the egg salad is high in fat. Choice **c** is incorrect. Peanut butter has a high fat content.

Category: Physiological Integrity: Basic Care and Comfort

Subcategory: Adult: Biliary Disorders

62. d. This client is exhibiting a somatic subtype of delusional disorder because he or she has an irrational belief that his or her body is either disfigured or nonfunctional. Choice **a** is incorrect. If the client had a conjugal delusion, he or she would have an irrational belief that his or her significant other is unfaithful. Choice **b** is incorrect. If the client were experiencing erotomania, he or she would have an irrational belief that someone with an elevated social status is emotionally or spiritually in love with him or her. Choice **c** is incorrect. If the client were experiencing a persecutory delusion she or he would have an irrational belief that there is a conspiracy against her or him.

Category: Psychosocial Integrity

Subcategory: Delusional Disorders

63. b. Clients diagnosed with Cushing's disease experience increased protein catabolism which results in a loss of muscle mass. As a result, supplemental protein is required. Choice **a** is incorrect. The client may be asked to restrict caloric intake to reduce weight. Choice **c** is incorrect. Fat intake should be restricted, but by more than 20%. Choice **d** is incorrect. The client should be encouraged to increase intake of potassium-rich food. This is because clients diagnosed with Cushing's disease often experience a low serum potassium level.

Category: Physiological Integrity: Basic Care and Comfort

Subcategory: Adult: Endocrine Disorders

64. The correct answer is 5, 6.

Clients with chronic pain physiologically adapt. As a result, the client will experience minimal changes in facial expressions and vital signs. Assessment findings such as elevated vital signs and facial grimacing are often experienced by a client in acute pain. Depression and physical inactivity are not physical assessment findings; however, some clients with chronic pain may report depression and physical inactivity.

Category: Physiological Integrity: Basic Care and Comfort

Subcategory: Adult: Pain Disorders

65. d. The client with gout should avoid foods that contain purines. Foods that are high in purines include: animal hearts, herring, mussels, yeast, smelt, legumes, sardines, and sweetbreads. Foods moderately high in purines include: anchovies, grouse, mutton, veal, bacon, liver, salmon, turkey, kidneys, partridge, trout, goose, haddock, pheasant, mushrooms, spinach, asparagus, cauliflower, and scallops. In addition, clients with gout should avoid beer and wine. Chocolate and milk do not contain purines.
Category: Physiological Integrity: Basic Care and Comfort
Subcategory: Adult: Musculoskeletal Disorders

66. a. This client may have complex underlying needs; a social worker must explore these needs and issues in order to provide the most appropriate interventions. Choice **b** is incorrect. Documenting the client's information is important, but doesn't ensure appropriate intervention. A social worker should be consulted. Choice **c** is incorrect. Although having the client discuss his or her feelings may be therapeutic, direct intervention to ensure the client's safety and well-being is most important. A social worker should be consulted. Choice **d** is incorrect. Offering the client the names and numbers of local shelters may be helpful, but the nurse isn't in a position to follow up on the client's care after discharge. A social worker should be consulted.
Category: Safe and Effective Care Environment: Coordination of Care
Subcategory: Adult: Mental Health Disorders

67. a. The nurse should encourage the mother to attend to the infant each time it cries to promote maternal infant bonding. Choice **b** is incorrect. Breast-feeding can promote maternal infant bonding. However, the mother and/or the infant may fall asleep during the feeding, increasing the risk of suffocation from the mother rolling onto the infant and the risk for Sudden Infant Death Syndrome from sleeping on a soft mattress with blankets and bedding. Choice **c** is incorrect. Maternal infant bonding will not be facilitated if the infant is in the nursery versus with the mother. Choice **d** is incorrect. The mother should use a soft, low-pitched voice to soothe the infant.
Category: Psychosocial Integrity
Subcategory: Maternal Infant: Neonate

68. d. It is recommended that the client attend 90 AA meetings in the first 90 days after a formal rehabilitation program. Choice **a** is incorrect. While the client should not drink at all, he or she will need help in staying alcohol-free after discharge and therefore should seek out a support system available through AA meetings. Choice **b** is incorrect. The client should not drink any type of alcoholic beverages. Choice **c** is incorrect. The client should avoid friends and situations that may trigger the client to use alcohol.
Category: Safe and Effective Care Environment: Coordination of Care
Subcategory: Adult: Mental Health Disorders

69. a. The nurse should assist the client when ambulating due to an increased risk for falls from adverse reactions to the medication, which include dizziness, hypotension, blurred vision, and lethargy. Choice **b** is incorrect. Coughing and deep breathing are encouraged after surgery and not indicated in this situation. Choice **c** is incorrect. While incontinence can be a side effect of benzodiazepines, the use of adult diapers may lead to skin breakdown. Choice **d** is incorrect. There is no indication that this client needs a vest restraint in this situation.

Category: Physiological Integrity: Risk Reduction

Subcategory: Mental Health: Medications

70. b. Listening to music or a radio show is the best recreational activity for a client who is newly blind. Choice **a** is incorrect. Listening to the television is inappropriate because it may cause the client anxiety since she can only hear and not see the television program. Choice **c** is incorrect. The client who is newly blind may not be ready to interact with other clients on the unit. Choice **d** is incorrect. This is inappropriate because the ability to read Braille is a learned skill.

Category: Safe and Effective Care Environment: Coordination of Care

Subcategory: Adult: Eye Disorders

71. d. The age of onset of puberty for boys is 13 to 15 years. Choice **a** is incorrect. The normal range for the onset of puberty in boys is 13 to 15 years of age. Choice **b** is incorrect. The nurse is able to address the parent's concern by stating that the normal range of puberty for boys is ages 13 to 15 years. Choice **c** is incorrect. This statement changes the focus from the client to the nurse, which is inappropriate.

Category: Health Promotion

Subcategory: Pediatrics: Adolescents

72. b. An occupational therapist helps people across the lifespan participate in the things they want and need to do through the therapy revolving around everyday activities. Common occupational therapy interventions include helping children with disabilities. The occupational therapist is most qualified to help a child with cerebral palsy eat and perform other activities of daily living. Choice **a** is incorrect. The occupational therapist is most qualified to help a child with cerebral palsy eat and perform other activities of daily living. Choice **c** is incorrect. While a social services professional might be useful for a child with cerebral palsy and his or her family, an occupational therapist is trained to help a child with such a condition eat and perform other activities of daily living. Choice **d** is incorrect. The occupational therapist is most qualified to help a child with cerebral palsy eat and perform other activities of daily living.

Category: Safe and Effective Care Environment: Coordination of Care

Subcategory: Pediatric Disorders

73. b. This is an example of late decelerations, that is, a drop in fetal heart rate after the peak of the contraction. Choice **a** is incorrect. Early decelerations occur before the peak of the contraction. Choice **c** is incorrect. A normal fetal heart rate forms a mirror image of the maternal contraction; as the contraction peaks, the fetal heart rate reaches its lowest point. Choice **d** is incorrect. In a variable deceleration, the fetal heart rate varies in onset, duration, and depth and may occur with contractions or between contractions.

Category: Safe and Effective Care Environment: Safety and Infection Control

Subcategory: Maternal Infant: Intrapartum

74. d. The infant should not be dusted with baby powder following a bath because this puts the infant at risk for developing pneumonitis secondary to aspiration of talc. Choice **a** is incorrect. A room temperature between 72 and 75 degrees F is appropriate. Choice **b** is incorrect. This is an appropriate method of checking the bathwater, as the elbow is very sensitive to temperature changes. Choice **c** is incorrect. This is appropriate mouth care for an 11-month-old infant.
Category: Safe and Effective Care Environment: Coordination of Care
Subcategory: Pediatric Disorders

75. b. The neonate with an Apgar score of 8 would require no interventions from healthcare professionals. Choice **a** is incorrect. The neonate would require gentle stimulation if the Apgar score were less than 8. Choice **c** is incorrect. The neonate would require oxygen if the Apgar score were less than 8. Choice **d** is incorrect. The neonate would require resuscitation if the Apgar score were between 0 and 3.
Category: Safe and Effective Care Environment: Safety and Infection Control
Subcategory: Maternal Infant: Neonate Assessment

76. d. The nurse should monitor the client's serum electrolytes. Hydrochlorothiazide is a potassium-depleting diuretic. The risk for digoxin toxicity increases when the serum potassium level is decreased. Choices **a, b,** and **c** are not as important as the serum electrolytes.
Category: Physiological Integrity: Pharmacology
Subcategory: Adult: Cardiac Disorders

77. d. The most appropriate information to share with the assistant is the procedure through which the spread of the HIV virus is controlled. Choice **a** is incorrect. This is an inappropriate statement and will not ease the assistant's concern. Choice **b** is incorrect. Although this information is true, it will not aid in easing the assistant's concern. Choice **c** is incorrect. Relaying how the virus is spread will not be useful in this situation. The most appropriate information to share is that which reinforces the way to control the spread of the HIV virus.
Category: Safe and Effective Care Environment: Coordination of Care
Subcategory: Adult: Immunological Disorders

78. b. The prone position is one in which the child would be placed on his or her abdomen. Choice **a** is incorrect. This is considered the Fowler's position. Choice **c** is incorrect. This is considered the supine position. Choice **d** is incorrect. This is considered the lateral position.
Category: Safe and Effective Care Environment: Coordination of Care
Subcategory: Pediatrics: Integumentary Disorders

79. c. The client will be instructed to take a side-lying position with his or her knees drawn up toward the chest. Or, the client may be instructed to sit on the edge of a chair or bed and lean forward over a table with the head and chest bent toward the knees. These positions help widen the spaces between the bones of the lower spine so that the needle can be inserted more easily. If fluoroscopy is used, the client would lie on his or her stomach so the fluoroscopy machine can take pictures of the spine during the procedure. Choices **a**, **b**, and **d** are incorrect. The client should be in the side-lying position with the knees drawn to the chest.
Category: Safe and Effective Care Environment: Coordination of Care
Subcategory: Adult: Neurological Disorders

80. d. The nurse should use an electric razor, not a standard razor, to avoid bleeding and injury. Choice **a** is incorrect. Preventing infection in this client population is a priority. Choice **b** is incorrect. The client's temperature should be taken orally or via the tympanic route versus rectally to avoid injury and bleeding. Choice **c** is incorrect. The client's teeth should not be cleansed with a toothbrush, which could cause injury and bleeding due to the brush's hard bristles.
Category: Safe and Effective Care Environment: Coordination of Care
Subcategory: Adult: Hematological Disorders

81. The correct answer is *startle* or *Moro reflex*. The neonate exhibits the Moro, or startle, reflex when he or she extends the arms and legs and then abducts them in response to a loud noise or being lowered suddenly.
Category: Health Promotion
Subcategory: Maternal Infant: Neonate Assessment

82. d. The nurse is aware that a sodium-restricted diet is prescribed to reduce the potential for excessive fluid volume and increased serum sodium levels. The most appropriate data to obtain to determine whether the client is having a therapeutic response to the low-sodium diet is daily weighing. Choice **a** is incorrect. The client's weight will change more than the client's skin turgor, especially day by day. Choice **b** is incorrect. The client's weight will change more than the client's pedal edema, especially day by day. Choice **c** is incorrect. Monitoring and documenting the client's sodium intake is an appropriate intervention. However, this does not provide the objective data provided by weighing the client daily.
Category: Safe and Effective Care Environment: Coordination of Care
Subcategory: Adult: Gastrointestinal Disorders

83. d. The wound, ostomy, continence (WOC) nurse is the most appropriate consult. The WOC nurse has specialty training in colostomy care. He or she will schedule a visit with a client who has a colostomy to offer support and provide teaching. Choices **a** and **b** are incorrect. The clinical nurse educator and the registered nurse do not have specialized training in ostomy care, even though either one could offer teaching at a later date. In this situation, the best option is the wound, ostomy, continence nurse. Choice **c** is incorrect. The social worker does not have specialized training in ostomy care. The social worker is trained in helping people solve and cope with problems in their everyday lives, making referrals, and so forth.
Category: Safe and Effective Care Environment: Coordination of Care
Subcategory: Adult: Gastrointestinal Disorders

84. d. Placenta previa, a condition in which the placenta partially or totally covers the maternal cervix, is a risk factor in preterm deliveries. Choice **a** is incorrect. Cervical incompetence is a risk factor for preterm delivery. Choice **b** is incorrect. Low socioeconomic status is a risk factor for preterm delivery. Choice **c** is incorrect. Implantation of the embryo into the uterine walls is essential if the pregnancy is to be maintained.
Category: Physiological Integrity: Reduction of Risk
Subcategory: Maternal Infant: Prenatal Complications

85. a. The client should avoid foods containing tyramine. Apples do not contain tyramine so the client does not need to avoid them. Choices **b**, **c**, and **d** are incorrect. Bananas, caffeine, and yogurt contain tyramine and should be avoided by the client taking Marplan.
Category: Physiological Integrity: Pharmacological Therapies
Subcategory: Mental Health: Medications

86. d. The physician obtains informed consent from clients. Informed consent is when permission is obtained from the client to perform a specific test or procedure after the client has been fully informed about the test or procedure and the risks and benefits associated with it. Choice **a** is incorrect. The nurse must understand that, legally, the client must be mentally competent to give informed consent for procedures. Choice **b** is incorrect. Only the physician can obtain informed consent. The professional nurse is involved in the informed consent process, but only as a witness to it and doesn't actually obtain the consent. Choice **c** is incorrect. The nurse should understand that only a minor who is married or emancipated can give informed consent.
Category: Safe and Effective Care Environment: Coordination of Care
Subcategory: Adult: Miscellaneous

87. d. A limb restraint is the best choice for this client. Applied to the wrists, limb restraints prevent the client from inadvertently dislodging the endotracheal tube. Choice **a** is incorrect. A belt restraint is often used to remind clients to stay seated in a wheelchair or seat. Choice **b** is incorrect. Four-points are typically only used temporarily during psychiatric emergencies. Choice **c** is incorrect. A vest restraint is often used to remind clients to stay seated in a wheelchair, seat, or bed.

Category: Safe and Effective Care Environment: Coordination of Care

Subcategory: Adult: Respiratory Disorders

88. a. Vitamin K should be administered by IM injection, not SQ. The preceptor should stop the LPN and have her reevaluate her injection method. Choice **b** is incorrect. The preceptor can distract the newborn, but she should first stop the nurse from administering the vitamin K by the wrong route. Choice **c** is incorrect. The nurse is not preparing to administer the injection correctly, therefore the preceptor must intervene. Choice **d** is incorrect. Vitamin K should be administered through an IM injection; the Z-track method is not indicated.

Category: Safe and Effective Care Environment: Safety and Infection Control

Subcategory: Adult: Pediatric Disorders

89. a. The child with severe gastroenteritis will experience diarrhea. The nurse should institute standard precautions to ensure other clients and healthcare providers are not put at risk for acquiring the infection. Choice **b** is incorrect. The client should be placed in a private room to avoid the spread of infectious body fluids. Choice **c** is incorrect. Gastroenteritis is severely contagious. The client should be provided with plastic utensils that will be discarded after meals, ensuring that the risk of transmission is decreased. Choice **d** is incorrect. The nurse should double-bag all the client's linens.

Category: Safe and Effective Care Environment: Safety and Infection Control

Subcategory: Adult: Pediatric Disorders

90. d. The parents should be told to keep the penis as dry as possible until the stent is removed. The child should not soak in a bathtub. Choice **a** is incorrect. This is an unnecessary action and may cause irritation to the penis. Choice **b** is incorrect. The client will not have a catheter in place. The child with a urinary stent is often sent home to void in a diaper. Choice **c** is incorrect. The client should be well hydrated following this procedure; fruit juice should not be avoided.

Category: Safe and Effective Care Environment: Safety and Infection Control

Subcategory: Adult: Pediatric Disorders

91. c. Using a bed alarm and moving the client to a room closer to the nurse's station is the most appropriate nursing action. The bed alarm will alert the nursing staff immediately if the client attempts to get out of the bed. Choice **a** is incorrect. Using all four side rails is considered a restraint and should be implemented as a last resort. Choice **b** is incorrect. A family member may choose to stay with the client, but it is inappropriate to expect or ask this of the family. Choice **d** is incorrect. This is an inappropriate nursing action that will interfere with the client's sleep patterns and privacy.

Category: Safe and Effective Care Environment: Safety and Infection Control

Subcategory: Mental Health Disorders

92. c. Irregular contractions are a sign of false labor. Choices **a**, **b**, and **d** are incorrect. Bloody show, contractions that increase with ambulation, and progressive dilation of the cervix are signs of true labor.

Category: Health Promotion

Subcategory: Maternal Infant: Intrapartum

93. c. Increased depression, not euphoria, can be a side effect of suddenly stopping an SSRI. Choices **a**, **b**, and **d** are incorrect. Constipation, diarrhea, and headaches can be side effects of stopping an SSRI suddenly.

Category: Physiological Integrity: Pharmacological Therapies

Subcategory: Mental Health: Medications

94. c. Motor vehicle accidents are the number-one cause of accidental injuries in high school students. Choice **a** is incorrect. While alcohol consumption is a growing problem with high school students, motor vehicle accidents are the number-one cause of high school accidental injuries. Choice **b** is incorrect. While domestic violence is a serious concern, it is not a cause of accidental injuries. Choice **d** is incorrect. Substance abuse is a growing problem in high school youth, but motor vehicle accidents are the number-one cause of accidental high school injuries.

Category: Physiological Integrity: Risk Reduction

Subcategory: Pediatrics: Adolescents

95. c. This is the most likely intervention to ensure the highest level of fall prevention. When the nursing staff makes rounds of the unit and clients' rooms the nurse is better able to identify at-risk situations. Choice **a** is incorrect. This action, placing a "Fall Risk" sign outside the client's room, may be helpful, but making rounds of the unit and clients' rooms provides the nursing staff an immediate opportunity to intervene and teach the client, family, and staff when a risk is noted. Choice **b** is incorrect. This action—wearing a color-coded armband—may be helpful, but making rounds of the unit and clients' rooms provides the nursing staff an immediate opportunity to intervene and teach the client, family, and staff when a risk is noted. Choice **d** is incorrect. This action—positioning the clients' beds in the lowest position—may be helpful, but making rounds of the unit and clients' rooms provides the nursing staff an immediate opportunity to intervene and teach the client, family, and staff when a risk is noted.

Category: Safe and Effective Care Environment: Safety and Infection Control

Subcategory: Adult: Miscellaneous

96. a. Completely emptying the breast at each feeding will decrease the risk for mastitis. Choice **b** is incorrect. Consistently feeding an infant on same breast will increase the risk for mastitis; breast milk may pool in the breast not used and thereby increase the risk for infection. Choice **c** is incorrect. Utilization of improper latching-on technique can lead to cracks and fissures on the nipples that can cause breast infection. Choice **d** is incorrect. Hand hygiene can reduce the risk for mastitis regardless of whether the mother utilizes hand sanitizer or soap and water.
Category: Safe and Effective Care Environment: Safety and Infection Control
Subcategory: Maternal Infant: Postpartum Complications

97. a. To obtain accurate readings, the nurse should recalibrate the machine whenever a new battery is installed. Choice **b** is incorrect. To adhere to standard precautions and prevent contact with blood, the nurse's hands should remain gloved throughout the entire blood glucose testing. Choice **c** is incorrect. The type of blood drop is determined by the type of strip the nurse is using: Some use a "hanging drop" of blood versus a small drop for strips that draw blood in with a capillary action. However, no matter which type of blood drop is indicated, the nurse should never smear the sample. Choice **d** is incorrect. The nurse should make sure the client's digit is dry prior to the procedure. The nurse will then wipe the selected area with an alcohol prep pad and wait until the alcohol evaporates.
Category: Safe and Effective Care Environment: Safety and Infection Control
Subcategory: Adult: Miscellaneous

98. d. The main route of transmission for hepatitis A is the fecal-oral route, rarely parenteral, that is, other than through the intestinal tract. If the client focuses on good hand hygiene before eating or preparing food, the client understands how to prevent transmission. Choice **a** is incorrect. Alpha-interferon is used in the treatment of chronic hepatitis B and C, not A. Choice **b** is incorrect. Using a condom during sexual intercourse is not a strategy to aid in preventing the spread of hepatitis A. Choice **c** is incorrect. Percutaneous transmission, that is, through the skin, is seen with hepatitis B, C, and D, not A.
Category: Safe and Effective Care Environment: Safety and Infection Control
Subcategory: Adult: Gastrointestinal Disorders

99. c. Medical asepsis requires infection control practices that reduce and prevent the spread of microorganisms. Objects are considered "clean," which means the absence of almost all microorganisms. Surgical asepsis is the elimination of all microorganisms, including pathogens and spores, from an area to render the area sterile. Cleansing the environment to prevent the spread of organisms is a form of medical asepsis. Hand washing is a technique used to prevent the spread of infection. The techniques illustrated in 3 and 4 are examples of surgical asepsis; they are activities a nurse would do to protect and maintain the sterile field.
Category: Safe and Effective Care Environment: Safety and Infection Control
Subcategory: Adult: Gastrointestinal Disorders AC

100. a. The priority is to help the girl find prenatal care to decrease the risk of complications. Choice **b** is incorrect. While helping the girl to quit drinking is important, the priority is to help the girl find prenatal care, because without it the adolescent and her unborn baby are at higher risk for complications. Choice **c** is incorrect. While helping the girl to quit smoking is important, the priority is to help the girl find prenatal care because without it the adolescent and her unborn baby are at higher risk for complications. Choice **d** is incorrect. While the nurse may want the girl to tell her parents about the pregnancy, it is the adolescent's right to decide whether to tell her parents. The priority is to help the girl find prenatal care because without it the adolescent and her unborn baby are at higher risk for complications.

Category: Physiological Integrity: Reduction of Risk

Subcategory: Pediatrics: Adolescents

101. c. The nurse finds the correct injection site by placing the palm of the hand on the greater trochanter and palpating the superior iliac spine with the index finger. The middle finger palpates the bony ridge of the iliac crest. The triangle formed between the index and middle finger is the site for the injection. Choice **a** is incorrect. This is too far laterally. Choice **b** is incorrect. The nurse does not use the site between the third and fourth fingers. Choice **d** is incorrect. The nurse does not use the site between the thumb and index finger.

Category: Physiological Integrity: Pharmacological Therapies

Subcategory: Maternal Infant: Medication

102. c. The client is utilizing the ineffective coping mechanism of distancing, which can occur when a client is unwilling or unable to discuss an event. Choice **a** is incorrect. Anxiety can be a symptom of a mental health disorder but it is not a coping mechanism. Choice **b** is incorrect. Depression can be a symptom of a mental health disorder but it is not a coping mechanism. Choice **d** is incorrect. Refusing care is not a coping mechanism but a right of the client. There is not an indication that the client is refusing care.

Category: Psychosocial Integrity

Subcategory: Mental Health: Coping Mechanisms

103. c. Choice **c** is correct. The palmar grasp reflex—involving all the fingers in grasping an object—should disappear around three months of age. Because it has not disappeared, the infant may need additional evaluation. Choice **a** is incorrect. The ability to build a 4-block tower does not normally occur until around 20 months of age: it is not expected in a 5-month-old. Therefore, this infant does not need additional evaluation. Choice **b** is incorrect. A 5-month-old infant should be able to grasp objects voluntarily. The infant is developing within the normal range and therefore does not need additional evaluation. Choice **d** is incorrect. The pincer grasp—involving the thumb and forefinger—develops around 8 to 12 months of age and therefore is not expected in a 5 month old infant. This infant does not need additional evaluation.

Category: Physiological Integrity: Reduction of Risk

Subcategory: Pediatrics: Infants

104. a. The nurse's priority/first action is to assess the client for injuries. Choice **b** is incorrect. The nurse completes an incident report; however, his or her priority responsibility is to assess the client for injuries. Choice **c** is incorrect. The nurse notifies the client's healthcare provider; however, his or her priority responsibility is to assess the client for injuries. Choice **d** is incorrect. The nurse may notify the nurse manager of the fall; however, his or her priority responsibility is to assess the client for injuries.
Category: Safe and Effective Care Environment: Safety and Infection Control
Subcategory: Adult: Musculoskeletal Disorders

105. d. The Rhogam is effective if the mother does not produce Rh antibodies. Choice **a** is incorrect. The fetus in not able to produce Rh antibodies. Choice **b** is incorrect. Rhogam impacts the mother's, not the fetus's, ability to produce Rh antibodies. Choice **c** is incorrect. The goal of Rhogam administration is to prevent the mother from producing Rh antibodies.
Category: Physiological Integrity: Pharmacological Therapies
Subcategory: Maternal Infant: Medication

106. b. Malpractice is a term used to describe negligence by a nurse; malpractice is professional negligence. Choice **a** is incorrect. Criminal negligence is when the crime falls outside the boundaries of a simple error and reflects a serious lack of concern for the safety of the client. Choice **c** is incorrect. A misdemeanor is a crime of lesser degree under the law and generally is punished by imprisonment for less than a year or a monetary fine. Choice **d** is incorrect. Tort is a civil wrong committed by one person against another.
Category: Safe and Effective Care Environment: Coordination of Care; Safety and Infection Control
Subcategory: Adult: Miscellaneous

107. b. Airway suctioning is always a nursing priority. The client who may experience respiratory/airway compromise should be attended to first. Choice **a** is incorrect. Airway suctioning is always a nursing priority. A dressing change, while important in the treatment of a wound, can be attended to after. Choice **c** is incorrect. Airway suctioning is always a nursing priority. Cleansing, while important to the comfort of the patient, can be attended to after. Choice **d** is incorrect. While a patient in need of medication for incisional pain is a priority, airway suctioning is always the highest nursing priority. The client who may experience respiratory/airway compromise should be attended to first.
Category: Safe and Effective Care Environment: Safety and Infection Control
Subcategory: Adult: Miscellaneous Disorders

108. The correct answer is *bargaining*.

Dr. Elisabeth Kubler-Ross's stages of grief and the order in which they occur are: denial, anger, bargaining, depression, and acceptance.

Category: Physiological Integrity: Basic Care and Comfort

Subcategory: Mental Health: Death and Dying

109. c. Prostaglandin E helps to ripen the cervix for delivery. Choice **a** is incorrect. Pain relief can be obtained from administration of epidural and intravenous medications, but not prostaglandin E. Choice **b** is incorrect. Prostaglandin E does not prevent cervical infections. Choice **d** is incorrect. Prostaglandin E does not prevent postpartum bleeding.

Category: Physiological Integrity: Pharmacological Therapies

Subcategory: Maternal Infant: Medications

110. c. Unlike a cooling sponge bath, where the temperature of the water begins at 90 degrees F and is gradually lowered to 65 degrees F at the end, the temperature for a tepid sponge bath starts and ends at 90 degrees F.

Category: Safe and Effective Care Environment: Safety and Infection Control

Subcategory: Adult: Miscellaneous Disorders

111. a. This is the correct location of the gallbladder. Choice **b** is incorrect. This is the liver. Choice **c** is incorrect. This is the pancreas. Choice **d** is incorrect. This is the stomach.

Category: Health Promotion and Maintenance

Subcategory: Adult: Gastrointestinal Disorders

112. a. Calcium gluconate is the antidote for magnesium sulfate toxicity. Choice **b** is incorrect. Methergine is used for postpartum hemorrhage. Choice **c** is incorrect. Narcan is used for opioid toxicity. Choice **d** is incorrect. Rhogam is used to prevent maternal Rh antibodies from forming when the mother is Rh negative and the fetus is Rh positive.

Category: Physiological Integrity: Pharmacological Therapies

Subcategory: Maternal Infant: Medication

113. b. The dorsal gluteal muscle—in the back of the hip—should not be utilized in the toddler. Choice **a** is incorrect. The deltoid—a muscle in the shoulder—is an appropriate choice in the toddler for some intramuscular injections such as the flu shot. Choice **c** is incorrect. The rectus femoris—a muscle in the thigh—can be used for intramuscular injections in the toddler. Choice **d** is incorrect. The vastis lateralis—a muscle in the thigh—can be used for intramuscular injections in the toddler.

Category: Physiological Integrity: Pharmacological Therapies

Subcategory: Pediatrics: Medication Administration

114. c. Manipulative behavior is one of the symptoms of antisocial personality disorder. Choice **a** is incorrect. Changes in appetite can be associated with mental disorders such as anxiety or depression, but not with antisocial personality disorder. Choice **b** is incorrect. Low energy levels can be associated with mental disorders such as depression, but not with antisocial personality disorder. Choice **d** is incorrect. Repetitive motions are a symptom of obsessive compulsive disorder.

Category: Psychosocial Integrity

Subcategory: Mental Health: Personality Disorders

115. c. Cephalohematoma is a swelling of the soft tissues between the bone and periosteum that does not cross the suture lines. Choice **a** is incorrect. Anencephaly is when the neonate is born without parts of the brain and/or skull. Choice **b** is incorrect. Caput succedaneum is a swelling of the soft tissues of the skull that crosses the suture lines. Choice **d** is incorrect. Dandy-Walker syndrome occurs when a section of the cerebellum is missing.
Category: Physiological Integrity: Physiological Adaptation
Subcategory: Maternal Infant: Neonate

116. d. This assessment indicates the nurse is assessing the posterior tibial pulse. Blood is carried to the posterior part of the leg and the foot's plantar surface via the posterior tibial artery. Choice **a** is incorrect. This illustration indicates the nurse is assessing the posterior tibial, not dorsalis pedis, pulse. Choice **b** is incorrect. This illustration indicates the nurse is assessing the posterior tibial, not femoral, pulse. Choice **c** is incorrect. This illustration indicates the nurse is assessing the posterior tibial, not popliteal, pulse.
Category: Health Promotion and Maintenance
Subcategory: Adult: Cardiovascular Disorders

117. c. Russel's sign is bruising of the knuckles, resulting from scraping as the hand is inserted in the mouth and rubbed against the teeth to induce vomiting, often found in clients with bulimia. Choice **a** is incorrect. Low self-esteem is a risk factor for anorexia. Choice **b** is incorrect. Model-child syndrome, or trying to be the perfect child, is a risk factor for anorexia. Choice **d** is incorrect. Sexual abuse is a risk factor for anorexia.
Category: Physiological Integrity: Reduction of Risk
Subcategory: Mental Health: Eating Disorders

118. a. The arm board should remain in place/position. Removing the arm board or untaping the arm board could dislodge the IV. Choice **b** is incorrect. Untaping the arm board could dislodge the IV. Choice **c** is incorrect. Removing the arm board could dislodge the IV. Choice **d** is incorrect. The arm board should remain in place.
Category: Health Promotion and Maintenance
Subcategory: Pediatrics

119. c. The nurse should instruct the client to report leg swelling, pain, redness, and/or warmth, which might indicate another pulmonary embolus. Choice **a** is incorrect. The client should elevate his or her legs, which promotes venous return to the heart. Choice **b** is incorrect. The client should not restrict fluids. Limiting fluids increases blood viscosity, which can promote clot formation. Choice **d** is incorrect. The client should ambulate daily.
Category: Health Promotion and Maintenance
Subcategory: Adult: Respiratory Disorders

120. b. The ultimate outcome for the client should be that she solves problems by herself, collaborating in her own care. Choice **a** is incorrect. While it is important that the client follow up with the psychiatrists, this will not ensure that the client will fully comply with the prescribed treatment and medication regimen. The ultimate outcome for the client is that she solves problems by herself, collaborating in her own care. Choice **c** is incorrect. The client's taking her prescribed medications alone will not ensure success unless the client knows how to address and solve problems without help from others. Choice **d** is incorrect. The client's understanding the side effects of her medications will not ensure success unless the client knows how to address and solve problems without help from others.
Category: Health Promotion and Maintenance
Subcategory: Mental Health Disorders

121. c. The fundus is at the level of the umbilicus at 20 weeks gestation. Choice **a** is incorrect. The fundus is below the level of the umbilicus until 19 weeks of gestation. At 20 weeks, the fundus is at the level of the umbilicus. Choice **b** is incorrect. This is too low. The fundus is at the level of the umbilicus at 20 weeks gestation. Choice **d** is incorrect. The fundus is above the umbilicus at 21 weeks gestation through delivery of the fetus.
Category: Physiological Integrity: Physiological Adaptation
Subcategory: Maternal Infant: Antepartum

122. a. Answer: 2 tablets
$$\frac{\text{desired} \times \text{tablet(s)}}{\text{available}} = \text{tablet(s) per dose}$$
$$\frac{5\text{ mg} \times 1\text{ tablet}}{2.5\text{ mg}} = 2\text{ tablets}$$
Category: Physiological Integrity: Pharmacology
Subcategory: Adult Cardiovascular Disorders

123. c. A head circumference of a neonate that is more than 3 cm larger than the chest circumference may be indicative of hydrocephalus. Choice **a** is incorrect. The swelling from caput succedaneum would not impact the head and chest circumference. Choice **b** is incorrect. The swelling from the cephalohematoma would not impact the head and chest circumference. Choice **d** is incorrect. Molding might be indicated if the head circumference was equal to or less than the chest circumference.
Category: Safe and Effective Care Environment: Coordinated Care
Subcategory: Maternal Infant: Neonate

124. a. The blood pressure will increase, not decrease, when experiencing anger because of the autonomic nervous system response to epinephrine secretion. Choice **b** is incorrect. Decreased peristalsis is an expected finding when a client is experiencing anger. Choice **c** is incorrect. Increased muscle tension is an expected finding when a client is experiencing anger. Choice **d** is incorrect. Increased respiratory rate is an expected finding when a client is experiencing anger.
Category: Psychosocial Integrity
Subcategory: Mental Health Disorders

125. b. This is the correct location to auscultate the apical pulse for a child under the age of 4. The heart's apex for a toddler is located at the fourth intercostal space immediately to the left of the midclavicular line. The heart of a child this age is more horizontal and larger in diameter than that of an adult. Choice **a** is incorrect. This is the location of the sternum. Choice **c** is incorrect. This is the area to auscultate the apical pulse in children age 4 to 6. Choice **d** is incorrect. This is where the nurse would auscultate the apical pulse in an adult.
Category: Health Promotion and Maintenance
Subcategory: Pediatrics

126. c. It is important to provide the client with a quiet room in which to sleep. Alcohol is metabolized in the body at a slow, steady rate. It is best to have the client sleep off the effects of the alcohol. Choice **a** is incorrect. The nurse does not need to have the client drink black coffee. The rate of alcohol metabolism is not influenced by caffeine. Choice **b** is incorrect. The nurse does not need to have the client take cold showers. The rate of alcohol metabolism is not influenced by taking a cold shower. Choice **d** is incorrect. The nurse does not need to have the client walk around the unit. The rate of alcohol metabolism is not influenced by ambulating.
Category: Psychosocial Integrity
Subcategory: Mental Health Disorders

127. c. Giving a young child aspirin when they have flulike symptoms or chicken pox increases the child's risk for Reye's syndrome. Choice **a** is incorrect. Aspirin does not increase the risk for appendicitis in children. Choice **b** is incorrect. Unless the child has a rare allergy to aspirin, it will not cause an asthma attack. Choice **d** is incorrect. Untreated strep throat increases the child's risk for rheumatic fever; aspirin does not.
Category: Physiological Integrity: Pharmacological Therapies
Subcategory: Pediatric: Medication

128. a. The nurse should ask the client whether he has a plan for killing himself because the more concrete the plan, the higher the risk for suicide. Choice **b** is incorrect. Asking the client whether he has a will does not help assess the risk for suicide. Choice **c** is incorrect. The nurse should not avoid talking about suicide as this will not help determine the client's risk for suicide. Choice **d** is incorrect. Telling the client that he has a lot to live for does not help determine the client's risk for suicide, which should be the nurse's priority in this situation.
Category: Physiological Integrity: Reduction of Risk
Subcategory: Mental Health: Suicide

129. b. Restating or rephrasing the mother's thoughts is the most appropriate and therapeutic response. This will provide the mother with an opportunity to express her thoughts further and for the nurse to offer clarification. Choice **a** is incorrect. This is a nontherapeutic response by the nurse, and can imply the nurse believes the mother is in some way to blame for the infant's illness. Choice **c** is incorrect. Telling the mother that the baby will be fine can offer the mother false reassurance. Choice **d** is incorrect. Even though this is a true statement, it ignores the mother's statement and does not provide her an opportunity to express her feelings.
Category: Psychosocial Integrity
Subcategory: Pediatric Disorders

130. b. The client's statement may indicate that the client's anxiety stems from her alteration in body image that often occurs following cardiac surgery. Choice **a** is incorrect. The client is not concerned about altered tissue perfusion; she is focusing on her body image. Choice **c** is incorrect. The client is focusing on body image, not her present hospitalization. Choice **d** is incorrect. Although the client may lack knowledge related to her postoperative course of care, in this instance she is focusing on her altered body image.
Category: Psychosocial Integrity
Subcategory: Adult: Cardiovascular Disorders

131. b. Encouraging the client to express his or her feelings is the most therapeutic response. This may also provide the nurse with the opportunity to provide the client with information that will aid in the coping process. Choice **a** is incorrect. This is a nontherapeutic response and ignores the client's statement and concerns. Postoperative teaching is an ongoing process and is completed by the entire healthcare team. Choice **c** is incorrect. This is a nontherapeutic response. The nurse should not assume the family will take care of the client. Choice **d** is incorrect. This is a nontherapeutic response and could actually block communication between the client and nurse and make the client hostile.
Category: Psychosocial Integrity
Subcategory: Adult: Vascular Disorders

132. d. The nurse understands that finding an alternative method of dealing with stress is the foundation of stress management. The use of relaxation techniques is highly recommended. Choice **a** is incorrect. Avoidance of stressful conversations will not necessarily reduce the client's stress. Choice **b** is incorrect. This is an unrealistic goal for the client. It is impossible to remove all stressors from one's life. Choice **c** is incorrect. Antianxiety medications are prescribed during acute periods of anxiety, but are not a routine part of a stress-reduction program.
Category: Psychosocial Integrity
Subcategory: Adult: Endocrine Disorders

133. c. The nurse should respond to the client based on the knowledge of dislocation precautions. These precautions include: avoiding extreme adduction (inward movement), internal rotation, and 90-degree flexion of the surgical hip for at least 4 to 6 weeks following surgery. Choice **a** is incorrect. Decreasing the use of the abductor pillow—one used to help spread the legs out—does not strengthen the hip muscles. Choice **b** is incorrect. This is a nontherapeutic response and does not address the client's concerns. Choice **d** is incorrect. Utilizing a cushioned toilet seat does not aid in the prevention of a dislocation of the prosthesis.

Category: Psychosocial Integrity
Subcategory: Adult: Musculoskeletal Disorders

134. c. Striking a tuning fork and placing it midline on the parietal bone to see whether the client hears it equally in both ears is how the Weber test is conducted. Choice **a** is incorrect. Standing 18 inches behind client and whispering a statement to test the client's ability to hear is not how the Weber test is conducted. Choice **b** is incorrect. Standing 18 inches in front of the client and whispering a statement is how the Whisper test, not the Weber test, is conducted. Choice **d** is incorrect. Striking a tuning fork and placing it on the mastoid process is the first step in the Rinne test, not the Weber test.

Category: Health Promotion and Maintenance
Subcategory: Adult: Assessment

135. d. A 10-week-old infant with pyloric stenosis will exhibit vomiting after feeding. Choice **a** is incorrect. Absence of the rooting reflex may be indicative of a neurologic dysfunction but not pyloric stenosis. Choice **b** is incorrect. Decreased suck reflex will impact the infant's ability to obtain food from the breast or bottle but it is not a symptom of pyloric stenosis. Choice **c** is incorrect. Spitting up after feedings is a common, normal occurrence in 10-week-old infants.

Category: Physiological Integrity: Physiological Adaptation
Subcategory: Pediatrics: Gastrointestinal Disorders

136. a. The priority for care is airway, bleeding, circulation (ABC), so the nurse's first action should be to check the client's airway patency. Choice **b** is incorrect. The nurse should follow the ABCs (airway, bleeding, circulation) for prioritizing care and check the client's airway patency and check for bleeding prior to checking the heart rate and blood pressure. Choice **c** is incorrect. The nurse should check the client's airway patency, then for bleeding, and then the heart rate to follow the ABCs (airway, bleeding, circulation) for prioritizing care. Choice **d** is incorrect. The nurse should follow the ABCs (airway, bleeding, circulation) for prioritizing care and check the client's airway patency, then for bleeding, and then the heart rate and blood pressure.

Category: Safe and Effective Care Environment: Safety and Infection Control
Subcategory: Adult: Postoperative

137. c. The normal range for sodium is 135 to 145 mEq/L. Choice **a** is incorrect. The normal range of blood urea nitrogen (BUN) values is 8 to 25 mg/dL. Choice **b** is incorrect. The normal range for fasting blood glucose levels is 70 to 125 mg/dL. Choice **d** is incorrect. The normal range for potassium is 3.5 mEq/L to 5.2 mEq/L.
Category: Safe and Effective Care Environment: Safety and Infection Control
Subcategory: Adult: Laboratory Values

138. a. Azelex is a topical medication used to treat acne. Choice **b** is incorrect. Azelex is a topical medication used to treat acne, not eczema. Choice **c** is incorrect. Azelex is a topical medication used to treat acne, not excessive hair growth. Choice **d** is incorrect. Azelex is a topical medication used to treat acne, not herpes simplex.
Category: Physiological Integrity: Pharmacology
Subcategory: Adult: Integumentary Disorders

139. c. Bronchovesicular breath sounds are auscultated in this area. These breath sounds have a medium pitch and intensity and are heard anteriorly over the mainstem bronchi on either side of the sternum and posteriorly between the scapulae. Choice **a** is incorrect. No breath sounds are auscultated in this area. Choice **b** is incorrect. Bronchial breath sounds are auscultated in this area. These breath sounds are loud and high-pitched. These breath sounds often resemble the sound generated when blowing through a hollow pipe. Choice **d** is incorrect. Tracheal breath sounds are auscultated in this area. These breath sounds are loud and high-pitched. They are heard over the trachea which is not routinely auscultated.
Category: Health Promotion and Maintenance
Subcategory: Adult: Respiratory Disorders

140. a. Following the steps of the nursing process, the nurse should assess, plan, implement, and evaluate care. Therefore the nurse should assess consciousness prior to implementing an intervention. Choice **b** is incorrect. Following the steps of the nursing process, the nurse should assess, plan, implement, and evaluate care. Therefore the nurse should assess consciousness prior to assisting the client back to bed. Choice **c** is incorrect. Following the steps of the nursing process, the nurse should assess, plan, implement, and evaluate care. Therefore the nurse should assess consciousness prior to calling the client's family. Choice **d** is incorrect. Following the steps of the nursing process, the nurse should assess, plan, implement, and evaluate care. Therefore the nurse should assess consciousness prior to calling the client's physician.

Category: Safe and Effective Care Environment: Safety and Infection Control
Subcategory: Adult: Falls

141. a. The nurse should place the child in the knee-chest position to promote venous return and decrease the child's cyanosis and dyspnea. Choice **b** is incorrect. The right lateral position will not promote the venous return that is needed to decrease the child's cyanosis and dyspnea. Choice **c** is incorrect. Standing will not promote the venous return that is needed to decrease the child's cyanosis and dyspnea. Choice **d** is incorrect. Placing the child in the Trendelenburg position—with head lower than the feet—will further increase the child's dyspnea and cyanosis.

Category: Physiological Integrity: Physiological Adaptation
Subcategory: Pediatrics: Cardiovascular Disorders

142. a. The nurse should utilize gloves and a gown—precautions used under contact isolation conditions—when caring for this patient. The nurse should also wash his or her hands with soap and water. A mask is not needed. Choice **b** is incorrect. The nurse should use a gown and gloves—precautions used under contact isolation conditions—but a mask is not needed. Additionally, the nurse should wash his or her hands with soap and water as hand sanitizer is not effective when a client has a C. diff infection. Choice **c** is incorrect. The nurse should also use gloves and a gown, but a mask is not needed when taking vital signs on a patient in contact isolation. Choice **d** is incorrect. The nurse should use soap and water to cleanse his or her hands as well as wear gloves and a gown, but a mask is not needed when taking vital signs on a patient in contact isolation.

Category: Safe and Effective Care Environment: Safety and Infection Control
Subcategory: Adult: Infectious Diseases

143. a. The client should limit/avoid canned vegetables due to their high sodium content. Choices **b**, **c**, and **d** are incorrect. Frozen fruits, lean meats, and low-fat yogurts are included on the DASH diet.

Category: Health Promotion and Maintenance
Subcategory: Adult: Cardiovascular

144. b. Donepezil (Aricept) is used in clients with Alzheimer's disease. Choice **a** is incorrect. The medication used to treat alcohol abuse is disulfiram (Antabuse). Choice **c** is incorrect. Antidepressants such as bupropion (Wellbutrin) are used to treat depression; donepezil (Aricept) is use to treat Alzheimer's disease. Choice **d** is incorrect. Antipsychotic medications such as Thorazine and Polixin are used to treat psychotic symptoms; donepezil (Aricept) is used to treat clients with Alzheimer's disease.

Category: Physiological Integrity: Pharmacological Therapies

Subcategory: Mental Health: Medications

145. d. The nurse should hold the digoxin and notify the physician that client's pulse rate is 45. Choice **a** is incorrect. The nurse should not administer the digoxin if the client's pulse is less than 50 beats per minute. Choice **b** is incorrect. The nurse should not administer the digoxin if the client's pulse is 50 beats per minute or less. Choice **c** is incorrect. The nurse should not administer the digoxin when the pulse rate is less than 50 beats per minute. Additionally, while a pulse rate of 45 is low, there is no indication that the patient is experiencing cardiac arrest at this time so it is not necessary to call a code.

Category: Safe and Effective Care Environment: Safety and Infection Control

Subcategory: Adult: Medication Administration

146. a. The tape measure should be placed across the eyebrows. Choice **b** is incorrect. Placing the tape measure at the hairline may lead to a smaller measurement. The nurse should place the tape measure across the infant's eyebrows. Choice **c** is incorrect. Placing the tape measure at the center of the forehead will lead to inaccuracy as different nurses will determine the center of the forehead differently. To standardize measurement technique, nurses should measure the head circumference by placing the tape measure over the eyebrows. Choice **d** is incorrect. Placing the tape measure over the infant's eyes will cause discomfort to the infant and will lead to an inaccurate measurement. The tape measure should be placed over the infant's eyebrows.

Category: Safe and Effective Care Environment: Basic Care and Comfort

Subcategory: Pediatrics: Infant

147. c. Fatal reactions may occur if sertraline (Zoloft) is administered at the same time as a monoamine oxidase inhibitor (MAOI) such as phenelzine sulfate (Nardil). The nurse should not administer the medications and should contact the physician. Choice **a** is incorrect. It is safe to take metformin (Glucophage) and phenelzine sulfate (Nardil) together. Choice **b** is incorrect. It is safe to take metformin (Glucophage) and sertraline (Zoloft) together. Choice **d** is incorrect. It is safe to administer phenelzine sulfate (Nardil) and cetirizine (Zyrtek) together.

Category: Safe and Effective Care Environment: Safety and Infection Control

Subcategory: Adult: Medication Administration

148. b. While there is no expiration date on a living will, general guidelines recommend that clients review their living wills annually. Choice **a** is incorrect. While the client may choose to review the living will every month, general guidelines are that living wills should be reviewed annually. Choices **c** and **d** are incorrect. While there is no expiration date on a living will, it is generally recommended that clients review their living will on an annual basis.

Category: Safe and Effective Care Environment: Coordinated Care

Subcategory: Adult: Advance Directives/Living Wills

149. a. The nutritionist would be involved to facilitate adherence to a consistent carbohydrate diet with increased protein to promote wound healing. Choice **b** is incorrect. Occupational therapists assist clients with fine motor movement. There is no indication that this client is having difficulty with fine motor movement. Choice **c** is incorrect. Recreational therapists assist clients with improving their emotional, mental, and physical health through activities. There is no indication that this client needs recreational therapy at this time. Choice **d** is incorrect. Risk managers are concerned with liability and potential lawsuits. There is no indication that a risk manager needs to be involved with this client.

Category: Safe and Effective Care Environment: Coordinated Care

Subcategory: Adult: Integumentary

150. c. Toe tapping is a symptom of akathesia, not drug-induced Parkinson's disease. Choices **a**, **b**, and **d** are incorrect. A flat affect, a shuffling gait, and tremors are symptoms of drug-induced Parkinson's disease.

Category: Physiological Integrity: Pharmacological Therapies

Subcategory: Mental Health: Medications

151. c. Café au lait spots are oval or round in shape and light brown in color. Choice **a** is incorrect. Bluish-black spots on the buttocks and sacrum are most likely Mongolian spots. Choice **b** is incorrect. A dark-red birthmark with an irregular border is most likely a port wine stain or a hemangioma depending on whether the birthmark increases in size. (Port wine stains do not increase in size; hemangiomas increase in size over time.) Choice **d** is incorrect. Tiny white sebaceous glands across the nose are most likely milia.

Category: Physiological Integrity: Physiological Adaptation

Subcategory: Pediatrics: Infant

152. a. Linea nigra is a benign dark line that runs down the center of the pregnant woman's abdomen. Choice **b** is incorrect. Melasma, also known as the mask of pregnancy, appears as blotchy hyperpigmented areas on the cheeks, nose, and forehead. Choice **c** is incorrect. Montgomery tubercles are enlarged sebaceous glands on the areola. Choice **d** is incorrect. Striae gravidarum are stretch marks that appear on the enlarging abdomen, breasts, thighs, and buttocks of the pregnant woman.

Category: Physiological Integrity: Basic Care and Comfort

Subcategory: Maternal Infant: Antepartum

153. b. The client should be placed in one-to-one observation to prevent another suicide attempt. Choice **a** is incorrect. Administering a sedative for sleep is inappropriate. Choice **c** is incorrect. There is no indication that the client needs isolation precautions at this time. Choice **d** is incorrect. Placing the client in a vest restraint is inappropriate at this time.
Category: Safe and Effective Care Environment: Safety and Infection Control
Subcategory: Mental Health: Suicide

154. c. The nurse should report to the ER and identify the tasks that he or she can safely perform and consult with the ER charge nurse/manager. Choice **a** is incorrect. The nurse cannot refuse an assignment or refuse to perform patient care, except that, in this situation, the nurse should identify the tasks that he or she can perform and notify the ER charge nurse/manager of these limitations. Choice **b** is incorrect. Contacting the hospital's vice president of nursing is not necessary in this situation. Choice **d** is incorrect. The nurse should identify which task he or she can safely perform versus simply performing the tasks typically assigned to a nursing aide. While it might be decided that the nurse would perform the duties of a nursing aide, this would only occur after the nurse met with the manager or charge nurse to identify tasks the nurse could safely perform.
Category: Safe and Effective Care Environment: Coordinated Care
Subcategory: Role of PN

155. d. This is the location of the anterior fontanel, a diamond-shaped wedge that if widened and bulging can indicate ICP. This is a common technique used to assess infants suspected of increased ICP. Choice **a** is incorrect. This is the location of the posterior fontanel. The posterior fontanel is usually closed and nonpalpable after the first 6 to 8 weeks of life. If it does not close, this could indicate underlying hydrocephalus or congenital hypothyroidism. Choice **b** is incorrect. This is the location of the sagittal sutures. Choice **c** is incorrect. This is the location of the coronal sutures.
Category: Health Promotion and Maintenance
Subcategory: Pediatrics

156. The correct answer is *peripheral artery disease (PAD).*
With peripheral artery disease, the client is experiencing decreased blood flow to the lower extremities; wrapping the extremities tightly with ace wraps would further decrease arterial blood flow to the extremities.
Category: Safe and Effective Care Environment: Coordinated Care
Subcategory: Adult: Circulatory

157. b. The child should be kept home from school until 48 hours after beginning treatment. This mother needs additional teaching. Choice **a** is incorrect. The mother should administer the eyedrops as ordered. No further teaching is indicated. Choice **c** is incorrect. Placing a cool compress to the child's eye is appropriate, therefore no further teaching is indicated. Choice **d** is incorrect. A separate towel and washcloth should be used for the infected child, therefore no further teaching is indicated.

Category: Safe and Effective Care Environment: Safety and Infection Control

Subcategory: Pediatrics: Head, Eye, Ear, Nose, and Throat (HEENT) Disorders

158. c. The client with GERD should eat small, frequent meals. Choices **a**, **b**, and **d** are incorrect. The client with GERD should avoid spicy foods, decrease caffeine intake, and sleep with the upper body elevated.

Category: Safe and Effective Care Environment: Coordinated Care

Subcategory: Adult: Gastrointestinal

159. b. Nodules noted at the distal interphalangeal joint (DIP), the joint closest to the fingertip or tip of the toe, that occur in clients with osteoarthritis are known as Heberden's nodes. Choice **a** is incorrect. Bouchard's nodules are noted in clients with osteoarthritis at the proximal interphalangeal joints, located in the middle of the fingers and/or toes. Choice **c** is incorrect. Hemangiomas occur as papules or raised, reddish or purplish areas of flesh. Choice **d** is incorrect. Mongolian spots appear as areas of dark-blue or purple discoloration on the buttocks of African American and Hispanic infants.

Category: Safe and Effective Care Environment: Coordinated Care

Subcategory: Adult: Musculoskeletal

160. a. The child should avoid products containing aspartame. Choices **b**, **c**, and **d** are incorrect. The child does not need to avoid broccoli, bananas, or fructose, but the child should avoid aspartame, meat, and dairy products.

Category: Safe and Effective Care Environment: Coordination of Care

Subcategory: Pediatrics: Endocrine Disorders

161. c. The nurse should administer the IM flu vaccine in the center of the deltoid muscle, approximately 2 to 3 finger widths below the acromial process. Choice **a** is incorrect. This position is posterior to the center of the deltoid. Choice **b** is incorrect. The position depicted is too close to the acromial process. Choice **d** is incorrect. The position depicted is anterior to the center of the deltoid.

Category: Safe and Effective Care Environment: Safety and Infection Control

Subcategory: Fundamentals of Care

162. The correct answer is *cerebellum*. The cerebellum controls balance as well as fine and gross motor functions.

Category: Safe and Effective Care Environment: Coordinated Care

Subcategory: Adult: Neurovascular

163. b. Women who do not breast-feed their children are at a higher risk for breast cancer. Choice **a** is incorrect. Age 13 is within the normal limits for having the first period. Women who had their first period earlier than age 11 are at increased risk for breast cancer. Choice **c** is incorrect. Women who have not had children are at higher risk for breast cancer. Choice **d** is incorrect. Women who do not exercise and are overweight are at increased risk for breast cancer.

Category: Physiological Integrity: Reduction of Risk Potential

Subcategory: Adult: Cancer

164. c. This is the client's sacrum. Choice **a** is incorrect. This is the client's left buttock. Choice **b** is incorrect. This is the client's right buttock. Choice **d** is incorrect. This is the client's gluteal fold.
Category: Physiological Integrity: Basic Care and Comfort
Subcategory: Adult: Integumentary

165. c. Hand hygiene before and after seeing each client is the best way to prevent the spread of nosocomial infections. Choice **a** is incorrect. While using a gown for patients in isolation can help reduce the spread of nosocomial infections, the best intervention is hand washing before and after seeing each client. Choice **b** is incorrect. While using gloves as part of universal precautions can help reduce the spread of nosocomial infections, the best intervention is hand washing before and after seeing each client. Choice **d** is incorrect. While using sterile technique for certain dressing changes can help reduce the spread of nosocomial infections, the best intervention is hand washing before and after seeing each client.
Category: Safe and Effective Care Environment: Infection Control
Subcategory: Adult: Miscellaneous Disorders

ADDITIONAL ONLINE PRACTICE

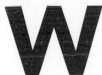hether you need help building basic skills or preparing for an exam, visit the LearningExpress Practice Center! On this site, you can access additional practice materials. Using the code below, you'll be able to log in and get additional practice. This online practice will also provide you with:

- **Immediate scoring**
- **Detailed answer explanations**
- **Personalized recommendations for further practice and study**

Log in to the LearningExpress Practice Center by using this URL: **www.learnatest.com/practice**

This is your Access Code: **9124**

Follow the steps online to redeem your access code. After you've used your access code to register with the site, you will be prompted to create a username and password. For easy reference, record them here:

Username: _____   **Password:** _____

With your username and password, you can log in and answer these practice questions as many times as you like. If you have any questions or problems, please contact LearningExpress customer service at 1-800-295-9556 ext. 2, or e-mail us at **customerservice@learningexpressllc.com**.

NOTES

NOTES